The Folk Remedy Handbook

Old-Fashioned Cures That Prevent and Reverse Pain, Obesity, Heart Disease, Cancer, Diabetes and More

By The Editors of FC&A Medical Publishing®

Publisher's Note

This book is intended for general information only. It does not constitute medical, legal, or financial advice or practice. The editors of FC&A have taken careful measures to ensure the accuracy and usefulness of the information in this book. While every attempt has been made to ensure accuracy, errors may occur. Some websites, addresses, and telephone numbers may have changed since printing. We cannot guarantee the safety or effectiveness of any advice or treatments mentioned. Readers are urged to consult with their professional financial advisers, lawyers, and health care professionals before making any changes.

Any health information in this book is for information only and is not intended to be a medical guide for self-treatment. It does not constitute medical advice and should not be construed as such or used in place of your doctor's medical advice. Readers are urged to consult with their health care professionals before undertaking therapies suggested by the information in this book, keeping in mind that errors in the text may occur as in all publications and that new findings may supersede older information.

The publisher and editors disclaim all liability (including any injuries, damages, or losses) resulting from the use of the information in this book.

My child, pay attention to what I say. Listen carefully to my words. Don't lose sight of them. Let them penetrate deep into your heart, for they bring life to those who find them, and healing to their whole body.
Proverbs 4:20-22

FC&A Medical Publishing®
103 Clover Green
Peachtree City, GA 30269
www.fca.com

Produced by the staff of FC&A
ISBN 978-1935574989

Table of contents

Allergies

Fight annoying allergies with 5 tasty foods

Stop suffering from allergies. You can find relief in your supermarket — no prescription necessary. Just make sure to eat plenty of apples, onions, oranges, peppers, and pineapples. These five foods are packed with natural antihistamines that treat allergy symptoms.

You're familiar with the usual signs of allergies — a stuffy or runny nose, sneezing, and itchy or watery eyes. Histamine is the bad guy that causes these reactions. It's an inflammatory chemical that battles infection as part of your body's immune response. Allergic reactions can stem from dust, animal dander, mold, pollen, or grass. Some foods — like nuts, shellfish, dairy products, or wheat — can also trigger allergy symptoms.

Antihistamine drugs can be costly and come with unwanted side effects, like sleepiness, dizziness, upset stomach, irregular heartbeat, and blurred vision. Rather than rely on them, try eating foods rich in the following two nutrients. They're natural, safer, and cheaper — and also much tastier.

Vitamin C. A natural solution for allergies, vitamin C seems to keep your white blood cells from releasing histamine and then neutralizes whatever histamine does appear. Research shows that your histamine levels rise when you don't get enough vitamin C. So eat peppers, citrus fruits like oranges, and other foods rich in this nutrient regularly. It works best when you get it all the time, not just when your allergies flare up.

Quercetin. Apples and onions provide plenty of quercetin, a flavonoid that fights inflammation and regulates histamine release. You can also find quercetin in broccoli, kale, scallions, berries, and tea.

To make quercetin even more effective, eat quercetin-rich foods with pineapple. This delicious tropical fruit contains bromelain, an enzyme that boosts quercetin's absorption. Bromelain also has anti-inflammatory powers that help combat allergies.

Keep these fantastic foods and nutrients in mind when you need to keep your allergies under control.

Watch out for allergy imposters

You tested negative for a particular allergy, but you get symptoms like diarrhea, hives, or sneezing whenever you eat, drink, or encounter your suspected allergen. Unfortunately, allergy antihistamines may not help your symptoms.

Food intolerance and nonallergic rhinitis produce the same symptoms as histamine-induced allergies, but they're caused by different processes in your body. With food intolerance, your digestive system doesn't have what it needs to digest a particular food. Nonallergic rhinitis symptoms occur because your immune system and mucous membranes grow more sensitive to irritants as you age.

Allergy antihistamines don't help either of these because histamine doesn't cause the symptoms. Look for anti-inflammatory nasal sprays or anticholinergic inhalers to ease nonallergic rhinitis, and talk to your doctor to find answers to food intolerance.

Battle wheezing and sneezing with beans

Do you have allergies or asthma? You could be low in one essential vitamin. Research from the Johns Hopkins School of Medicine explains why tasty foods like beans may help. Folate seems to be the key.

When scientists examined the medical records of more than 8,000 participants in a national health and nutrition survey, they found an interesting occurrence. People with the lowest blood levels of this B vitamin had a 40 percent higher risk of wheezing and a 31 percent higher risk of allergies than those who had the highest blood levels of folate.

> If you have allergies or wheezing, that may be a sign you need to include extra folate in the menus you prepare.

People lacking folate also had higher levels of Immunoglobulin E (IgE) antibodies. Your body's immune system makes these antibodies whenever it detects a foreign invader like an allergen. The more you produce, the more likely you'll react to an allergy-causing substance. The antibodies trigger the release of inflammatory chemicals, like histamine, that cause your allergy symptoms.

The Johns Hopkins scientists concluded that the more folate people had in their system, the lower their risk of wheezing, allergy symptoms, and high IgE levels. They suspect folate may help reduce allergic reactions by making positive changes to your immune system. Folate may also help prevent wheezing by fighting the inflammation that helps cause it.

Folate levels in your blood rise and fall with the amount of folate in your diet. An easy way to keep it up is with beans. They're high in folate, low in cost, and easy to add to your diet. Try to include beans or other folate-rich foods in at least one meal every day. Here are some good ways to start.

- Breakfast — For a little extra folate, eat like the British. Warm up canned baked beans, and spread them on lightly buttered toast. For a lot more folate, choose a breakfast cereal like Total Raisin Bran, Wheaties, or Special K.
- Lunch — Add a healthy dose of canned chickpeas (garbanzo beans) to a lunch salad, or enjoy soup with added lentils.
- Supper — Include a side of black-eyed peas or enriched rice, or make a main course of pinto bean, black bean, or kidney bean chili.

HEALTH ALERT!

Bacon lovers, beware. If you're allergic to cats, you may also find yourself reacting badly to pork. A rare double allergy called pork-cat syndrome has been discovered in the United States. It is caused by the albumin in cat saliva, cat dander, and pork products.

Symptoms vary widely but usually occur after eating pork. Examples include itching or swelling of the mouth, lips, or tongue; hives; and even life-threatening reactions that cause your windpipe to close up and blood pressure to drop dangerously low.

Many people allergic to cats are not allergic to albumin. But if you have a cat allergy and experience symptoms after eating pork, talk to your doctor. Medical help is available to treat and prevent the problem.

Reel in more allergy relief

A delicious seafood supper may do more than satisfy your appetite. It may also help your hay fever or skin allergies.

Experts suspect two omega-3 fatty acids in fish, eicosapentanoic acid (EPA) and docosahexaenoic acid (DHA), may help your body fend off an allergic reaction. Two studies show why they may be right.

Lower antibody levels. German researchers studying 388 people found that nearly 25 percent had Immunoglobulin E (IgE) antibody levels that suggested a high sensitivity to allergens. And in fact, interviews revealed that a significant number of study participants had been troubled by hay fever, allergic skin reactions, or symptoms of asthma.

But women who ate the most fish or consumed the most DHA had the lowest IgE levels, meaning less vulnerability to allergens. Oddly enough, the amount of fish men ate didn't make a difference. Researchers suspect this is because women have more estrogen in their bodies, and some studies suggest added estrogen may help the body convert fatty acids from foods into DHA.

Fend off hay fever symptoms. Another German study found that people who had more EPA and DHA in their red blood cell membranes had less risk of hay fever. The risk of hay fever also dropped as the amount of alpha-linolenic acid (ALA) in their diets rose. Although the study population didn't eat much fish, it did eat plenty of foods containing ALA, which your body converts to EPA.

> A fish or shellfish allergy doesn't have to keep you from the benefits of DHA and EPA. Instead, enjoy nuts and seeds rich in alpha-linolenic acid (ALA).

Benefit from natural anti-inflammatories. Your body produces IgE antibodies in response to substances your immune system identifies as dangerous. Although allergens aren't really dangerous, your body responds as if they are. The IgE antibodies latch onto mast cells in your nose, eyes, lungs, and digestive system, the places where people experience allergy symptoms. Then the IgE antibodies trigger the release of inflammatory chemicals from the mast cells to neutralize the allergen "threat."

Unfortunately, those chemicals trigger your allergy symptoms. But EPA and DHA are anti-inflammatory, so they interfere with the chemicals that cause your symptoms — and may even block the production of IgE antibodies in the first place.

To add more omega-3s to your diet, enjoy fatty fish like salmon, sardines, herring, rainbow trout, barramundi, and light canned tuna, or foods like flaxseed, almonds, pumpkin seeds, and walnuts. Just remember to take the precautions described in "4 things you should know before eating fish" in the *Rheumatoid arthritis* chapter.

HEALTH ALERT!

Your choice of beverage could make your allergy symptoms worse. Beer, wine, and liquor contain the same histamine that triggers hay fever symptoms like sneezing, coughing, itching, and headaches. Wine and beer also contain sulfites, another trigger for allergy and asthma symptoms.

One study suggests the risk of hay fever symptoms may nearly double for women who have two drinks a day compared with those who have less than one drink a week. So avoid beer, wine, and liquor when allergy symptoms are bothering you, and you may start feeling better.

Alzheimer's & memory loss

Cinnamon: Nature's astounding memory booster

Cinnamon seems simple enough. It perks up pies and spices up hot cocoa. And this humble spice in your kitchen cupboard may be on the cutting edge of Alzheimer's prevention.

Studies suggest that cinnamon may provide a clue to stopping Alzheimer's disease (AD). That's because certain components of cinnamon appear to block the formation of the brain plaques and tangles associated with AD.

- Israeli researchers conducted studies using cinnamon bark extract, and these studies yielded some promising results. In mice, the cinnamon extract inhibited the formation of amyloid-beta fibers. In test tubes, it broke up these dangerous proteins that can kill brain cells.
- Further studies involved fruit flies and mice genetically altered to give them Alzheimer's disease. Some of them received the cinnamon extract in their drinking water. Flies with AD normally have shorter life spans and impaired movement, but the flies treated with cinnamon extract lived about as long and climbed up a test tube about as well as healthy flies. Similarly, mice whose water contained the cinnamon extract improved their performance on memory tests. Their brains also showed reduced amyloid-beta deposits.

- In lab studies of human brain cells, University of California, Santa Barbara researchers found that cinnamon extract inhibited the buildup of tau, the protein that forms tangles in the brain. Preventing the formation of these tangles may be the key to stopping AD.

Proanthocyanidins, which are polyphenols found in cinnamon, and cinnamaldehyde, a major component of cinnamon's essential oil, likely both contribute to cinnamon's powers. Although proanthocyanidins act as antioxidants, it seems that something besides their antioxidant properties helps them fight tau buildup.

Much more research is needed, but these studies are a good start. Just don't start gobbling cinnamon by the spoonful. You'd need to eat a ridiculous — and toxic — amount to reap the benefits discovered in these studies. But keep your eyes open. Scientists may find a way to incorporate cinnamon extract into a useful treatment.

> Cinnamon can do more than help prevent AD. A dash of this spice only costs a few pennies, and it may help you avoid heart disease risk factors like high cholesterol and obesity.

In the meantime, it can't hurt to add a little more cinnamon to your diet. Sprinkle some on your oatmeal or breakfast cereal or stir it into a cup of tea.

Curry combats dementia

Multitasking is a must in today's fast-paced society — and eating curry is one delicious way to multitask. You get to enjoy a spicy, flavorful meal while keeping dementia at bay.

Curry powder, a blend of spices including turmeric, does quite a bit of multitasking in the fight against Alzheimer's disease (AD). Credit goes to curcumin, the polyphenol that gives turmeric its distinctive yellow color.

"We accidentally found out that it blocks every single step in Alzheimer's," says UCLA researcher Sally Frautschy.

That's important because the development of AD involves several factors. Accumulation of amyloid-beta plaques, the formation of tangles of tau protein, oxidative damage, and inflammation act individually or together to cause damage to brain cells and mental impairment. Rather than target just a single component, curcumin helps counteract all of them.

Here's a quick look at how curcumin helps protect your brain.

Breaks up brain plaques. Medical researchers found that folks in northern India had the lowest rate of Alzheimer's in the world. Was the curry in their diets fending off dementia? Maybe so. In the lab, the spices in curry powder not only stopped new brain plaques, they even weakened existing ones.

Curcumin did the job on new and already formed amyloid-beta plaques in both lab and animal tests. Some studies show that curcumin also thwarts the buildup of tau protein. These results suggest that turmeric, thanks to curcumin, is the one spice that can stop brain plaque from forming, putting the brakes on Alzheimer's.

Squelches inflammation. Unusual or chronic brain inflammation likely plays a role in AD. Curcumin's anti-inflammatory powers make it an ideal antidote. So be sure to add curry powder to pilafs and vegetables. This spice also goes great with deviled eggs, and chicken and lamb dishes.

Prevents oxidative damage. Curcumin has potent antioxidant activity, which led to its use as a food preservative. This antioxidant ability can also safeguard your brain from harmful free radicals.

Further research should shed more light on how curcumin works — and how to get the most out of it. But because of its many positive effects on brain health, curcumin could become a safe, effective treatment for Alzheimer's disease.

Until then, feel free to eat more curry and other foods, like yellow mustard, that feature turmeric. You can find turmeric in the spice aisle of your local supermarket. Add it to your dishes for extra flavor — and extra protection against dementia.

Fatty fish fights Alzheimer's

Afraid of losing your memories? Reel them back in with fish.

Fatty fish — like salmon, mackerel, and herring — is the main source of docosahexaenoic acid (DHA), an omega-3 fatty acid key to brain health. People who eat foods rich in DHA are nearly 40 percent less likely to develop Alzheimer's disease (AD).

Try the ultimate lube job for your brain

Fatty fish are a staple of the Mediterranean diet, an eating plan that's known to slow brain changes associated with the early development of dementia. The plan includes olive oil, which is great for boosting your memory.

In a small study, scientists asked 110 seniors to follow the Mediterranean diet for a year. However, half of the people were asked to replace all the vegetable oils they used with olive oil.

Researchers tested people's cognitive abilities before and after the trial and found that those who ate olive oil every day showed more improvement. That may be because the nutrients in olive oil helped fight inflammation and oxidative stress in the brain that can cause cognitive decline.

Want to try it yourself? People in the study ate about 1 1/2 to 2 1/4 tablespoons of olive oil a day. And they used extra-virgin olive oil, which contains more nutrients than light, or refined, olive oil.

That's what researchers at Tufts University discovered. The study involved 899 men and women from the large, ongoing Framingham Heart Study who did not have dementia at the study's onset. Their average age was 76, and the average follow-up was just over nine years.

The people with the highest blood levels of DHA were 47 percent less likely to develop dementia of any kind and 39 percent less likely to develop Alzheimer's disease compared to those with lower DHA levels. Not surprisingly, the people with the highest DHA levels also ate more fish. They averaged nearly three servings a week.

Just over half of the people in the study — 488, to be exact — also completed a food frequency questionnaire. Those who reported eating more than two servings of fish a week reduced their risk of developing dementia by 39 percent and slashed their risk of developing Alzheimer's disease by 50 percent compared to those who ate, at most, two servings of fish a week.

What makes DHA so important? You've heard the expression, "You are what you eat." That's especially true for your brain, where DHA is the most abundant fatty acid. Within the brain, DHA is especially prevalent in the gray matter that deals with memory, language, and thinking. It may protect you by reducing inflammation or blocking the buildup of brain proteins associated with AD.

Boost your defense against dementia by boosting your intake of DHA. You can do that by simply adding more fatty fish to your diet. Besides salmon, mackerel, and herring, good options include:

- tuna
- shad
- whitefish
- trout
- sardines
- sablefish
- bass
- pompano
- bluefish
- oysters
- halibut
- cod

Berries boost your brainpower

Is there really a food that can help you feel younger physically and mentally? Yes, according to some studies. And that's "berry" good news for your brain.

Berries may be small, but they can make a big impact on brain health. Chock-full of antioxidants, these tiny treats fight oxidative damage and inflammation, fending off a variety of age-related conditions, including Alzheimer's disease.

Black raspberries are loaded with nutrients you need for a better memory. But if you can't find them at the store, don't worry. You'll still be able to power up your brain with blueberries, which also have lots of antioxidants. You can't go wrong with strawberries, prunes, and blackberries, either.

Researchers have demonstrated that blueberry and strawberry extracts can reverse brain aging and memory deficits in rats. Human studies have also been promising.

- One small study found that blueberry juice gives your memory a boost. Nine people in their 70s with early memory decline drank the equivalent of about 2 1/2 cups of wild blueberry juice every day for 12 weeks. Not only did their ability to learn and recall information improve, they also experienced fewer symptoms of depression and lowered their blood sugar levels.
- Another study found that regularly eating strawberries may slow mental decline in women as they age.

Spark brain cells. Credit goes to anthocyanins, the flavonoids that give berries their vivid colors. Anthocyanins can cross the blood brain barrier. Once there, they may enhance brain cell connections, improve communication between cells, and stimulate brain cell regeneration. Researchers speculate a link between anthocyanins and the activation of signaling proteins through a specific pathway in the hippocampus, the brain region that controls learning and memory.

Remove toxic debris. A study suggests that berries may work in other ways, too. Blueberry and strawberry extracts helped microglia, the brain's housekeeping cells, do their job. Normally, microglia remove toxic debris from the brain in a process called autophagy. But with age, microglia become less effective and debris builds up, interfering with brain function. In the study, the berry extracts blocked a protein that shuts down the autophagy process, so order was restored.

You don't need to splurge on fancy, exotic berries like goji, noni, or acai. Everyday berries boost your blood levels of antioxidants just as much — but cost less. Black raspberries, blackberries, red raspberries, blueberries, and strawberries should all give you great bang for your buck.

To get the most benefits, opt for fresh or frozen berries rather than jams, jellies, or juice drinks. That way, you get more fiber and nutrients — without the added sugar and calories.

Hang on to memories with apple juice

As a child, perhaps you played tag in your yard, then quenched your thirst with a glass of apple juice. Now that you're older, something more dangerous may sneak up on you — like Alzheimer's disease (AD). But apple juice, the go-to beverage of your childhood, can still come in handy. Make an effort to outrun senility and Alzheimer's. Just sip two glasses a day of this drink for a month.

Safeguard memories. Researchers at the University of Massachusetts Lowell conducted a series of animal studies that suggest apple juice has brain-boosting powers. Here's a quick look at some of their findings.

- Mice who received the equivalent of two glasses of apple juice a day for a month produced less beta-amyloid, the protein responsible for forming plaques in the brains of people with AD.
- Apple juice helps maintain acetylcholine levels in aging mice. A key neurotransmitter, it's required for good memory, and low levels have been linked to Alzheimer's disease. Not surprisingly, the aging mice who got apple juice also performed better on maze tests.
- Aging mice whose diet included apple juice had less oxidative brain damage than mice given a standard diet. They were given the human equivalent of 2 to 3 cups of apple juice or two to four apples a day.

Antioxidants, including quercetin and other flavonoids, in apples and apple juice likely deserve the credit. But some other component of apple juice could also contribute to its success.

However it works, apple juice can be a healthy addition to your diet. It may spark fond memories of childhood — while making sure you don't lose those memories.

Boost declining moods. Even if a loved one already has Alzheimer's, apple juice can help. A study found that it improved the mood and behavior of 21 nursing home residents with moderate-to-severe AD. People in the study, who ranged in age from 72 to 93, received two 4-ounce glasses of apple juice each day for a month.

Although there were no changes in mental performance or the ability to perform day-to-day tasks, caregivers reported a 27-percent improvement in mood and behavior. Specifically, residents demonstrated less anxiety, apathy, agitation, depression, and delusion.

Whether you're trying to stave off Alzheimer's or slow its progression, try drinking more apple juice — the "kids' drink" with grown-up benefits.

Secret to a smarter coffee break

Eat a cookie during your next coffee break. You'll give your taste buds — and your brain — a treat. That's because the combination of caffeine and sugar helps your brain work more efficiently.

Spanish researchers found that people who received caffeine and glucose, a form of sugar, performed just as well on tests measuring attention and memory as those who received a placebo or either caffeine or glucose alone. However, MRIs of their brains showed reduced activity in the brain regions associated with these tasks. In other words, their brains worked just as well but didn't have to work as hard.

Caffeine and glucose seem to work together, so each substance enhances the effect of the other. Combining coffee with a sweet snack, like a cookie, could be an easy — and tasty — way to boost your brainpower.

Keep your wits with cantaloupe

Bigger doesn't always mean better. But a big, juicy cantaloupe may be one of your best bets to fend off mental decline. It's the biggest, cheapest fruit you're not eating but should be.

That's because cantaloupe is chock-full of beta carotene. This carotenoid, which your body converts to vitamin A, acts as a powerful antioxidant. Just a cup of cantaloupe balls gives you 3,575 micrograms of beta carotene and a whopping 120 percent of your daily requirement of vitamin A.

Here's what research says about beta carotene and your brain.

- The Physicians' Health Study II, which followed nearly 6,000 men age 65 or older, found that beta carotene supplements may guard against mental decline — but only with long-term use. Men who took beta carotene supplements for 15 years or more had slightly higher scores on memory tests, but those who took the supplements for three years or less showed no benefit. Although the differences were small, even very modest differences in memory can lead to big differences in the risk of developing dementia.

> If you're feeling exotic, reach for a mango, the tropical fruit that helps you think more clearly as you age —thanks to the 921 micrograms of beta carotene it provides.

- A UCLA study determined that high blood levels of beta carotene may protect against mental decline in older people who carry a certain gene that makes them more susceptible to Alzheimer's disease (AD).

So just how does beta carotene help? It likely works in two ways.

- As vitamin A, it normalizes the way your body processes beta-amyloid protein. A breakdown in this process is one culprit behind AD.

- As an antioxidant, beta carotene seems to boost brain function and brain cell survival as well as improve communication between brain cells. It may also make your brain more resistant to the toxic effects of beta-amyloid buildup in cells.

Eating more cantaloupe is one way to boost your beta carotene levels. But that's not the only reason to eat this sweet, delicious fruit. It's low in calories but high in nutrients. While a cup of cubed cantaloupe contains only 54 calories, it provides plenty of vitamin C, potassium, dietary fiber, and B vitamins, including niacin, vitamin B6, and folate. Add some cantaloupe to your fruit salad or just enjoy it on its own.

Other good — and good-tasting — sources of beta carotene include sweet potatoes, spinach, apricots, carrots, sweet red peppers, broccoli, and green leafy veggies like kale, collards, and turnip greens.

Beef up your brain with B12

It may sound like a low-budget horror movie — "The Incredible Shrinking Brain" — but brain shrinkage, or atrophy, is a seriously scary problem. If you have low levels of vitamin B12, you can be at greater risk for brain shrinkage and cognitive problems. That's because when you lose brain volume, you also lose essential thinking skills. Even healthy people experience some brain atrophy as they age, but it happens much more quickly for those with Alzheimer's disease (AD).

About 1 in 6 people over age 70 have mild cognitive impairment, and half of them develop AD. During this transition, brain atrophy occurs more quickly. Fortunately, vitamin B12 may be able to slow this decline.

This vital nutrient, also known as cobalamin, is found mostly in animal protein, including fish, meat, liver, poultry, milk, and eggs, giving more importance to the classic question, "Where's the beef?" Lean beef, as a good source of vitamin B12, can help keep your senses sharp.

A Rush University study involved 121 people ages 65 and older from the south side of Chicago. Researchers drew blood to measure vitamin B12 levels as well as markers that indicate B12 deficiency.

When these markers — including homocysteine and methylmalonic acid — were high, the news was not good. Total brain volume, as measured by MRI scans, was smaller and cognitive test scores were worse.

British researchers reported similar results. In a two-year study, B vitamins — including vitamin B12 — helped lower homocysteine, an amino acid produced by your body that can damage blood vessels. They also dramatically slowed the rate of brain atrophy in older folks with mild cognitive impairment. High levels of homocysteine have been linked to a higher risk of dementia, including Alzheimer's disease, and to brain atrophy.

In this Oxford University study, which included 168 people ages 70 and older, 85 people took B vitamins and 83 took a placebo. The B vitamin group received 0.8 milligrams (mg) per day of folic acid, 0.5 mg per day of vitamin B12, and 20 mg per day of vitamin B6.

Overall, the B vitamin group had a 31.7 percent lower concentration of homocysteine compared to the placebo group, and a nearly 30 percent lower rate of atrophy. For people with higher levels of homocysteine to start with, the results were even more impressive — their rate of brain atrophy was 53 percent lower than those in the placebo group.

Do you ever experience forgetfulness, numbness and tingling in your arms or legs, and confusion? Those are signs of a vitamin B12 deficiency.

More research is certainly needed, but these promising results indicate that boosting your vitamin B12 intake may help slow the development of Alzheimer's disease.

Stick to fish, lean beef and poultry, and low-fat dairy products for the healthiest sources of vitamin B12. For vegetarians or vegans, supplements are your best option.

Beet juice beats dementia

Looking to stay sharp as you age? Drink some beet juice, an unusual but delicious beverage that boosts your brainpower.

A Wake Forest study shows that beet juice increases blood flow to the brain. More specifically, it increases blood flow to the white matter of the brain's frontal lobes, regions often affected by cognitive decline and dementia.

> Watch out for one strange — yet harmless — side effect of drinking beet juice. You might end up with red stools or urine, a condition called beeturia.

When these areas don't get enough blood and oxygen, it can affect your memory and hamper your ability to perform daily tasks, like writing a check, using appliances, and shopping. Drinking beet juice could be an easy way to keep your brain in tiptop shape.

That's because beet juice provides plenty of nitrates. When you consume nitrates, good bacteria in your mouth convert them to nitrites, which help expand blood vessels to improve blood flow. Better yet, nitrites seem to target areas that need blood and oxygen. So they increase blood flow exactly where it's needed most.

In the Wake Forest study, 14 people over 70 were randomly assigned to either a high-nitrate or low-nitrate diet. The high-nitrate diet featured more vegetables — including spinach, lettuce, broccoli, and beet juice — while the low-nitrate diet contained few fruits and veggies but lots of grains, meats, and dairy products. Each diet provided the same amount of calories.

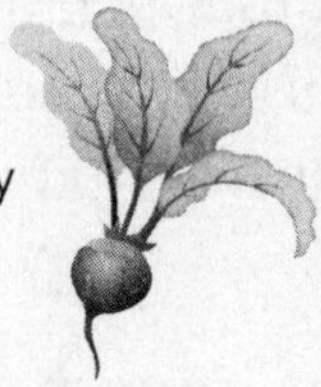

You don't need to get your beets in liquid form. Enjoy these colorful vegetables in a variety of ways. Try baking, roasting, steaming, boiling, grilling, or even pickling beets.

You don't even have to cook them. Shredded raw beets make a fine addition to any salad. Beet leaves are also edible. Use these tasty greens as you would Swiss chard or spinach.

In the supermarket, look for round, smooth, firm beets with a deep red color. Store them, unwashed, in the refrigerator for up to four weeks. Remove the more perishable greens first, though, and use them within four days.

When handling beets, you may want to wear rubber gloves. Otherwise, you could be caught red-handed. If your fingers or cutting boards turn red from beet juice, remove the stains with a mixture of lemon juice and salt.

On the first day, people ate their assigned breakfast, lunch, and dinner. On the second day, one hour after breakfast, they underwent an MRI to measure blood flow to the brain. For the third and fourth days, the two groups switched diets and repeated the MRI.

Regardless of the order, the high-nitrate diet led to increased blood flow to the white matter of the brain's frontal lobes. That suggests that boosting your nitrate intake may help boost your defense against mental decline.

Researchers note that the two diets likely provided different amounts of antioxidants and phytochemicals, so something besides the nitrates could be at work. But these results add to the possible benefits of beet juice. Previous studies have shown that beet juice lowers blood pressure and helps people exercise longer.

Look for beet juice, also known as beetroot juice, in health food stores. Or make your own with a juicer. You can mix it with other juices, like apple, carrot, or pineapple, according to your taste. The Wake Forest researchers developed a tastier beet juice by adding small amounts of sugar, citric acid, cranberry powder, and other additives.

Besides beets, you can also get nitrates from celery, cabbage, spinach, and some lettuce.

Wise up with water

Thirsting for the secret to a superior brain? Tap into the pure simple healing power of water. Just drinking water can boost your alertness, mood, memory, and decision-making ability. It's an easy way to give your brain a tuneup.

You need water to keep your brain — and the rest of your body — running smoothly. When you become dehydrated, your brain doesn't work as well. You don't have to run a marathon or work construction for hours in the hot sun to become dehydrated. It's surprisingly easy to do.

The dangers of dehydration. Losing just 2 percent of your weight from water loss can affect the way you think, feel, and act. Tests showed that people suffering this degree of dehydration scored lower on math skills, lost short-term memory abilities, were slower to make decisions, and were generally more fatigued than people with plenty of water to drink. Other studies have shown that drinking water makes people feel more alert, while dehydration worsens their moods and increases confusion.

Water is, in fact, so important to brain function that a person's hydration status needs to be considered during tests for dementia, stroke, and learning disabilities. That's because this deficiency could cause memory loss and make it seem like you have Alzheimer's.

A boost to your brain. Why does water make such a big splash in your brain? When you're dehydrated, water moves out of your cells to your bloodstream in an attempt to keep your blood volume and your blood pressure at a safe level. If dehydration continues, your cells shrivel up and no longer work properly. Your brain cells are particularly at risk since your brain is about 70 percent water. In addition, a lack of adequate water affects your blood brain barrier (BBB). This layer of cells and tissue separates your brain from the rest of your body, protecting it from foreign or dangerous substances in your blood. When you become overheated, without enough fluids to cool your body down, your BBB develops leaks, and that's bad news for your brain function.

So drink plenty of water throughout the day — even when you're not thirsty. As you age, your sense of thirst may diminish, but that doesn't mean you don't need water. Aim for between six and eight 8-ounce glasses a day. Keep in mind you may need even more water when exercising or dealing with hot temperatures

Eggs give your brain an edge

Scrambling for a nutritious way to help your brain? Eat more eggs. They are a good source of choline, an essential nutrient needed to produce the neurotransmitter acetylcholine. Low levels of this key brain messenger have been linked to memory loss and Alzheimer's disease. While some studies show that certain forms of choline may help improve mental function in people with Alzheimer's, other research has not been as promising.

In any case, boosting your intake of choline-rich foods, like eggs, should help keep your acetylcholine levels adequate — and your brain running smoothly.

How much choline do you need? Men should strive for at least 550 milligrams (mg) per day, while women should aim for at least 425 mg daily. But don't go overboard. You shouldn't get more than 3.5 grams of choline in one day.

To increase your choline intake, get cracking. One large egg provides 126 mg, mostly in the yolk. Poach, boil, or bake your eggs as a healthier alternative to frying them.

Besides meat and poultry in general, other good food sources of choline include:

- beef and chicken liver
- wheat germ
- shiitake mushrooms
- soybeans
- sun-dried tomatoes
- beans
- cod
- salmon
- peanut butter
- shellfish
- pistachios
- cauliflower

Protect your brain with purple veggie

You may find eggplant appealing — but if you want to retain its brain-boosting benefits, don't waste time peeling.

Babaganoush

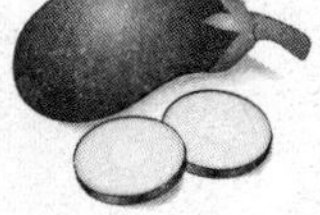

Puree roasted eggplant with garlic, tahini, lemon juice, and olive oil to make homemade babaganoush, a flavorful Middle Eastern spread.

Eggplant skin contains a mighty anthocyanin called nasunin. Anthocyanins give eggplants their deep purple color. But nasunin, a powerful antioxidant, does so much more.

- Researchers at the University of California at Berkeley found that nasunin protects brain cell membranes from damage. Specifically, it guards against lipid peroxidation, the process by which harmful free radicals steal electrons from the lipids, or fats, in cell membranes. You need healthy cell membranes to keep out free radicals, let in nutrients, and receive instructions from messenger molecules.
- In a later study, Japanese scientists discovered that nasunin also inhibits angiogenesis, or the growth of new blood vessels. While angiogenesis is important during the brain's development, it also contributes to tumors, the wet form of age-related macular degeneration, and possibly Alzheimer's disease. In fact, angiogenesis may help cause the leaky blood brain barrier seen in the brains of people with Alzheimer's.

The combination of its antioxidant powers and its ability to thwart angiogenesis could make nasunin — and, hence, eggplant — a beneficial brain food.

Just make sure to keep the skin on. After all, that's where the nasunin is. You should also try preparing healthy eggplant dishes. While eggplant parmesan may be delicious, it's also fried, breaded, and covered with layers of cheese.

Consider baking, roasting, steaming, or grilling eggplant. It makes a wonderful side dish or a welcome addition to salads or stir-fries.

When shopping, look for firm, smooth, shiny eggplants that are heavy for their size. The stem and cap should be bright green,

HEALTH ALERT!

Eggplant is not for everyone. As a member of the nightshade family — along with tomatoes, potatoes, and peppers — it could trigger an allergic reaction in some people. If you are allergic to latex, you may be sensitive to eggplant. It also contains chemicals called salicylates, which may cause trouble for some with a low tolerance for them.

Symptoms of a salicylate allergy include trouble breathing, headache, stuffy nose, itching, skin rash, hives, stomach pain, and swelling of your hands, feet, and face. In extreme cases, people with the allergy can experience anaphylaxis, a potentially deadly reaction that includes a drastic drop in blood pressure, loss of consciousness, and organ failure.

while the skin should be free of scars, bruises, and other marks. Store eggplant in the crisper of your refrigerator.

To tenderize this vegetable and make it taste less bitter, use this technique. Cut the eggplant into slices, then sprinkle them with salt. Let the slices sit for about half an hour to draw out some moisture. Then rinse off the salt and pat them dry.

Healthy diet leads to a healthy brain

Memory loss and Alzheimer's disease may be scary — but they're not inevitable. In fact, an analysis of studies estimates that about half of Alzheimer's disease cases could be prevented by lifestyle changes and treatment or prevention of chronic conditions.

Factors like diabetes, high blood pressure, obesity, smoking, depression, lack of mental activity, and a sedentary lifestyle increase your risk for Alzheimer's disease. But you can take steps to change each of them. Quit smoking, start exercising, challenge your mind, and get treatment for any medical conditions.

You can also fight off mental decline with your knife and fork. A healthy diet can keep your weight, blood pressure, cholesterol, and blood sugar levels under control — and keep your brain razor-sharp for years to come. For your brain and all-around health, try these tips.

Fill up on fruits and veggies. They provide plenty of antioxidants, including vitamins and phytochemicals, to fight dangerous free radicals.

Go fish. You'll get plenty of anti-inflammatory omega-3 fatty acids by eating fatty fish twice a week.

Fix the fat. Opt for olive or canola oil rather than butter, margarine, or other oils.

Boost your B vitamins. Low levels of folate, vitamin B6, and vitamin B12 lead to higher levels of harmful homocysteine and an increased risk of Alzheimer's disease. You can find B vitamins in whole grains, legumes, seeds, seafood, and dark leafy greens.

Don't forget about vitamin D. Studies show that low blood levels of vitamin D boost your risk for mental impairment. You can get vitamin D from food sources like fortified low-fat milk, eggs, liver, and sardines, as well as from sunlight and supplements.

Spice it up. Add zing to your dishes with brain-boosting spices like turmeric and cinnamon.

Anxiety & stress

Soothe stress with dark chocolate

You can build resistance to all kinds of stress, even if you often feel more anxious than the people around you. Best of all, a study from Europe suggests chocolate can help.

Swiss scientists tested 30 people to determine their stress levels. All 30 people were then assigned to eat a half bar of dark chocolate twice a day for two weeks. At the beginning, middle, and end of the study, the researchers took blood and urine samples from each participant to determine how the dark chocolate was affecting their body chemistry.

People who were highly stressed benefited the most from eating the chocolate. By the end of the study, their levels of stress hormones, like cortisol and catecholamines, had dropped. What's more, their stress-related changes to energy metabolism and gut microbes had improved, too.

Keep in mind this study was sponsored by the chocolate maker, Nestle. Although more research is needed, if you want to try dark chocolate, take the same approach as the people in the study.

- Choose a dark chocolate bar with a high cocoa content. You may need to read a few labels to find one.
- Make sure you limit yourself to 1 1/2 ounces a day.
- Read the label to determine fat grams and calories. Subtract similar amounts of fat and calories from elsewhere in your diet so you don't gain weight.

Once you have done that, enjoy the advantages dark chocolate has to offer. Not only does it provide healthy plant compounds called flavonoids, you'll also get some theobromine and caffeine that may stimulate you with a quick burst of energy. So be sure to savor half the bar as a midmorning pick-me-up, and enjoy the other half during your mid-afternoon slump. You'll be glad you did.

Did you know?

Just as the friendly probiotic bacteria in yogurt can help prevent diarrhea from antibiotics, French researchers say similar probiotics may help you put the brakes on stress. After scientists tested the stress and anxiety levels of 55 people, they instructed them to take a daily supplement for one month. Half the group took Probio'Stick, a product containing 3 million colony-forming units of the probiotics *Lactobacillus helveticus* and *Bifidobacterium longum*. The other study participants took a placebo.

Testing after the study found that people who had taken probiotics had lower anxiety scores than people who took a placebo. What's more, their stress hormone levels had dropped during the study, while the levels of the placebo group had not changed. Although Probio'Stick was not available in the United States when the study was published, other probiotic products that fight stress are now readily available in this country.

Relieve anxiety with fish

Just because you can't stop the stress in your life doesn't mean you have to live with the misery. A study suggests you can face the same level of stress every day, but feel less anxiety.

Ohio University researchers tested 68 medical students to determine their stress levels. During the following three months, half the students took a daily supplement containing omega-3 fatty acids, while the other half took a placebo. By the end of the study, students who took omega-3s saw their anxiety symptoms drop by 20 percent.

Omega-3s may help because anxiety is associated with an increase in cytokines in your body. Cytokines are compounds that promote inflammation. Fortunately, two omega-3 fatty acids, eicosapentaenoic acid (EPA) and docosahexaenoic acid (DHA), can help by raising your body's levels of inflammation-fighting compounds to help counteract these inflammation promoters.

EPA and DHA are found in fatty fish that live in cold water, but they can also be found in supplements like the one taken by the medical students. That particular supplement contained 2,085 milligrams (mg) of EPA and 348 mg of DHA. This may be why the students who took the omega-3 supplement not only had less anxiety, but also lower levels of inflammation than people who took the placebo.

> Next time you feel overwhelmed, munch on celery. This tasty veggie is loaded with phytochemicals that may reduce the amount of stress hormones in your body. These compounds could also improve your blood pressure.

Although the students took about five times as much EPA and DHA as you would normally get from fish, the researchers do not recommend you start taking fish oil capsules. Instead, they suggest getting more omega-3 fatty acids from your diet. Eating cold-water fatty fish twice a week may be the best way to start. Keep in mind some fish can give you a lot more EPA and DHA than others, so be picky. Choose fish like salmon, herring, whitefish, sardines, and lake trout.

If you are not satisfied with the results you get from eating fish more often, talk with your doctor before you try fish oil supplements. These supplements may not be safe if you have certain health conditions or take certain medications.

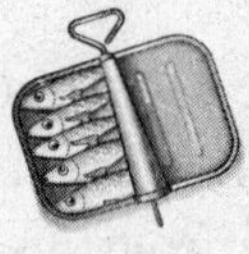

You may hesitate to eat fish because you worry that preparing fresh fish may require more time, energy, or effort than you can afford. To speed things up, start with canned sardines, canned tuna, or canned salmon.

For example, you can easily whip up a quick sandwich spread by mashing canned sardines and mixing them with Dijon mustard and minced onions. Just pay close attention to the labels on canned fish. Here are several good reasons why.

- Many brands contain added ingredients, like salt, that you don't want.
- Canned salmon may contain fish bones and skin unless you find "boneless" and "skinless" on the label.
- Some canned tuna contains high amounts of mercury. Stick with light tuna, the safest kind. Many experts recommend eating no more than 12 ounces a week.
- Make sure salmon labels promise that it is "wild."

Bacterial & fungal infections

Fight the superbug threat

Enjoying a daily cup of tea or coffee may be your ticket to avoiding a severe — and possibly deadly — infection. More than 250,000 people were hospitalized in one year alone by antibiotic-resistant infections — all caused by a microbe called methicillin-resistant *Staphylococcus aureus* (MRSA). Your risk of developing this infection may rise significantly if MRSA sneaks in and settles down in your nasal passages.

But a study from the Medical University of South Carolina found that people who drank hot tea or hot coffee were less likely to carry MRSA in their noses, as some 2 million people do. The researchers are not sure why this happens, but both beverages contain their own arsenals of antimicrobial compounds. Glyoxal, diacetyl, trigonelline, and methylglyoxal are the tough-sounding compounds that fortify coffee's arsenal, while tea fights back with tannic acid and catechins. In addition, both tea and coffee limit your body's ability to absorb iron, a mineral MRSA needs to grow.

If you happen to prefer cold tea, you won't see the same benefit. The researchers found iced tea did not protect against MRSA. Sodas didn't either. It could be that you breathe in the antimicrobial compounds when you sip beverages that are hot, or perhaps fewer antimicrobial compounds can survive in colder temperatures.

More research is needed to find out exactly why the noses of hot tea and coffee drinkers seem resistant to MRSA. Meanwhile,

Did you know?

Around 40 to 60 percent of women get a urinary tract infection (UTI) in their lifetime. And 1 in 4 suffers a repeat infection, made more likely if you've gone through menopause. That's because you have less good bacteria to combat the ones that cause infections. The key to protecting yourself may be in what you drink.

Fortunately, green tea may help you battle bad bacteria and prevent UTIs. Researchers at Oakland University William Beaumont School of Medicine examined the effects of green tea extract on UTI-causing bacteria — specifically *E. coli.* They found the polyphenols in green tea, especially epicatechin-3-gallate, kept the bacteria from growing. Drinking just 1 cup of green tea could positively affect the bacteria in your urinary tract, and several cups throughout the day could provide long-lasting protection.

experts say drinking a cup or two each day may help. You can even choose caffeinated or decaf since caffeine doesn't seem to affect the results. While you're at it, take these other essential steps to defend yourself against MRSA infections.

- Wash your hands, or use alcohol-based hand sanitizers regularly — especially after playing with pets or cleaning up after them, and when leaving a doctor's office, hospital, school, or any crowded place.
- Avoid letting your pets lick you.
- Keep cuts, scrapes, and wounds covered with a clean, dry bandage. Practice proper wound treatment and care until the damage heals.
- Do not share soap, towels, razors, or anything else that comes into contact with another person's skin.

- Clean your gym bag and athletic gear regularly. Promptly wash workout clothes after wearing.
- Bathe daily and after you exercise in case MRSA has gotten on your skin. Give your pets regular baths, too.

Amazing remedy provides sweet relief

Mary had been suffering from a painful leg ulcer for two weeks when she visited her doctor. For a couple of months, they tried treatment after treatment, but nothing helped. Meanwhile MRSA was discovered in the wound, and the pain was excruciating. So Mary and her doctor decided to try a different therapy.

Instead of taking antibiotics, Mary applied a dressing of specially prepared honey to the ulcer each day, covering it with a fluid-retaining bandage. The honey did what antibiotics and other medicine could not. In just three weeks, the MRSA was gone, and Mary's stubborn ulcer had healed completely.

Of course, this wasn't just any honey. It was manuka honey from New Zealand and Australia. This sweet treat has turned out to be surprisingly effective against antibiotic-resistant bugs like MRSA.

- Irish researchers discovered MRSA lurking in the venous leg ulcers of 16 people. Ten were treated with manuka honey and six with hydrogel medicine. After four weeks, manuka honey eliminated MRSA in seven out of 10 people treated with it. But only one of the six people treated with hydrogel got rid of MRSA.
- Sometimes MRSA or other infectious bacteria grow in a form called biofilm, a common cause of chronic sinus infections. These biofilms can be drug resistant. But a laboratory study found that manuka honey was better at killing MRSA biofilms and other biofilms than the antibiotics usually prescribed.

- Welsh researchers discovered that MRSA treated with manuka honey loses its FabI protein. This vital protein helps create the fatty acids needed to build cell walls and other cell structures. Without this protein MRSA cells cannot reproduce and eventually die.

The Irish and Welsh studies were not done with regular store-bought honey or even manuka honey purchased through the internet. The research was done with medical-grade manuka honey. That is important for two reasons:

- Store-bought honey has antibacterial properties, but manuka honey has extra microbe-fighting power.

- Regular honey is heat-treated to get rid of any microbes that could cause infection, but that may remove its antibacterial powers. Medical-grade manuka honey is sterilized with gamma radiation. This kills the clostridium spores that could cause an infection but does not affect the antibacterial powers of the honey.

If your doctor says you have a MRSA skin or wound infection, or if you have an infection that has become more swollen, red, and painful in spite of antibiotic treatment, ask your doctor whether medical-grade manuka honey could be right for you.

HEALTH ALERT!

An irritating boil, pimple, "spider bite," or lesion has appeared on your skin for no apparent reason. Don't just ignore it. You may have a possible MRSA skin infection. Don't touch or treat it yourself. Make an appointment to see your doctor as soon as possible. If a skin problem or recent wound becomes swollen, painful, red, or filled with pus, or if you develop a fever, see your doctor immediately.

Diet tricks to banish yeast infections

You may have more power to prevent yeast infections than you think. After all, yeast infections don't just happen. Something causes them — and it may be something you can control.

Recurring yeast infections are sometimes a sign of an undiagnosed condition, such as diabetes. Consult your doctor if you get them often. However, if he finds no underlying health concerns, changing your diet may help.

Search out the sugar. Yeast infections are caused by a fungus called *Candida albicans*, which needs certain ingredients to help it thrive. For example, *Candida* yeasts positively adore sugar. That may be why some studies suggest reducing the sugar in your diet to help prevent yeast infections. Why? Because when you eat less sugar, the *Candida* get less sugar, too. In fact, some experts think they have discovered which foods help *Candida* multiply like crazy. They suggest that you may feel better if you avoid the following foods:

- simple sugars like table sugar, corn syrup, and refined sugar as well as foods that contain these sugars, like soft drinks, fruit juices, and baked goods
- dairy products
- foods with high yeast content, including peanuts, mushrooms, cheese, dried fruit, leavened bread, and alcoholic beverages
- processed or refined foods, such as frozen dinners and chips
- foods made with white flour like white bread and pastries

Limit the oils. Some experts even recommend avoiding fruit, nuts, and foods that contain hydrogenated or partially hydrogenated oils. But once you start feeling better, a leading authority says, you can eat a less restricted diet.

Focus on helpful foods. This doesn't mean you are left with nothing to eat in the meantime. Foods that may help your body defend itself against *Candida* include:

- chicken, turkey, and eggs.
- fresh vegetables and vegetable pastas.
- whole grains like brown rice, or grain substitutes like buckwheat or quinoa.
- seafood.
- herb teas.
- seeds.
- oils like unrefined flaxseed or olive oil.
- yogurt with live and active cultures, or a probiotic supplement. The evidence for yogurt preventing yeast infections is mixed, so you can talk to your doctor about a probiotic supplement if you prefer to play it safe.

According to the Mayo Clinic, no clinical trials — the gold standard of studies — have shown that this diet can help. But while doctors at the Mayo Clinic may not be convinced this diet kills *Candida*, they also point out that it may help you feel better by cutting out processed foods that are high in calories and low in nutritional value.

Did you know?

You just picked up a new prescription for an infection and are greeted with a "horse pill." If you don't think you can swallow it without choking and gagging, try this easy trick to help the medicine go down. Turn your head to the left or right and then take the pill.

Bladder cancer

Single mineral helps sidestep disease

A selenium shortage could set you up for several deadly diseases. Studies have linked low selenium levels to lung, prostate, and digestive cancers. Now you can add bladder cancer to the list.

Researchers combed through the results of seven studies on selenium and bladder cancer. Overall, they found that people with the highest levels of this trace mineral were nearly 40 percent less likely to develop the disease. Women seemed to benefit more than men, maybe because their bodies process selenium a little differently.

Your body uses this mineral to build selenoproteins, which double as antioxidants. They mop up harmful compounds called free radicals before they can wreak any cancer-causing havoc. Selenium may also help repair the genetic material inside cells and make cancerous cells self-destruct.

Ideally, experts say, you should have 80 to 95 micrograms of selenium per liter of blood to maximize its cancer-fighting power. Your doctor can check your levels if you're concerned.

Most people get plenty of this mineral from their food. Cover your bases by loading your plate with healthy grains like barley, fish such as light or yellowfin tuna, and lean meats like turkey. It's possible to get a toxic dose of selenium from supplements, so talk to your doctor before taking them.

Sip your way to better health

Something as simple as drinking more water each day could prevent bladder cancer.

More than 47,000 men took part in the Health Professionals Follow-Up Study over the course of 22 years. Those who drank at least 2.5 liters (about 10 cups) of water or other fluids each day were 25 percent less likely to develop bladder cancer, compared to men who drank less than 1.3 liters (about 5 cups) a day.

Scientists suspect that fluids help flush out cancer-causing compounds before they can harm the cells that form the lining of your bladder — damage that can set the stage for cancer.

Men in this study drank less fluid, especially water, as they aged. Don't let this happen to you. Fill a pitcher with water and pop it in your refrigerator to chill overnight. Then drink it throughout the day.

Little-known danger from meat and fish

Eating a lot of red meat can increase your risk of bladder cancer, according to a study. "It's well known that meat cooked at high temperatures generates heterocyclic amines (HCAs) that can cause cancer," says Dr. Jie Lin, one of the study authors and assistant professor at the University of Texas M.D. Anderson Cancer Center.

HCAs form when high heat causes the protein in beef, pork, poultry, and fish to interact with creatine, a chemical naturally stored in the meat. Experts found that people who ate the most red meat were almost twice as likely to get bladder cancer, compared to those who ate little.

Cooking method matters most. All meats had an effect, depending on how they were cooked. Even chicken and fish raised the risk if they were fried. But beef steaks, pork chops, and bacon had the greatest impact on bladder cancer. So did the level of doneness. A preference for well-done meats nearly doubled the risk.

Genetics play a part. Some people react worse to HCAs than others. Their genes make them even more sensitive to the cancer-causing tendency of these compounds. Out of this group, those who ate the most red meat were up to five times more likely to develop bladder cancer.

You don't have to give up burgers and steaks entirely. It's easy to cut down on HCAs by changing the way you prepare your food. For more information about reducing HCAs naturally, see "Safer ways to eat red meat" in the *Prostate cancer* chapter.

Humble veggie boosts odds of survival

Just when you thought broccoli couldn't get any better, scientists say it could actually help you survive bladder cancer. It packs a satisfying crunch along with a wallop of anti-cancer compounds called isothiocyanates. These powerful compounds:

- help produce enzymes that clean up cancer-causing toxins.
- block cancer cells from maturing and multiplying.
- trigger cancer cells to self-destruct, a process known as apoptosis.

Amazingly, these compounds keep doing their job even after they have been cycled through your body and flushed out in your urine. In fact, being dissolved in urine gives them direct contact with your bladder walls, where they actively fight cancerous cells.

This could give new hope to people with bladder cancer. The disease is notoriously hard to beat, coming back in more than half of the people who undergo treatment. And if the cancer moves beyond surface cells in the bladder and attacks the muscle, the outlook gets worse.

Gives you an edge. Researchers questioned 239 people about the foods they typically ate before they were diagnosed with bladder cancer. People who ate as little as 1/2 cup of broccoli each month were less likely to die from the disease. Cooked broccoli dropped the risk by one-third. Raw broccoli slashed it by more than half.

No other cruciferous vegetable had as much of an impact. Maybe that's because broccoli boasts 40 percent more isothiocyanates than cabbage and 230 percent more than cauliflower, two vegetables in the same family.

Fresh is best. Cooking destroys some of these precious, anti-cancer compounds. That's why the raw vegetable had the greatest effect. Even though protection started with just 1/2 cup serving of raw broccoli a month — don't stop there. The top eaters in this study averaged four servings a month.

Simple spice crushes cancer

Can't stand broccoli? No worries. Mustard seed powder contains some of the same cancer-fighting compounds, and it's probably in your spice rack right now.

Cruciferous vegetables contain a type of isothiocyanate called allyl isothiocyanate (AITC). They aren't, however, the only sources. Hot, spicy seasonings such as mustard, horseradish, and wasabi are chock-full of AITC, too. This compound is what gives them their strong, sharp flavor.

The plants that go into making these spices store AITC in the form of sinigrin. When you chop up, chew, or grind them, the sinigrin turns into AITC.

> Smokers, in particular, could benefit from more broccoli. Smoking is the single biggest risk factor for bladder cancer. Broccoli isothiocyanates are especially good at neutralizing the cancerous compounds in cigarettes.

Studies show that the AITC you get from food eventually ends up in your urine. While that urine sits in your bladder, this compound goes to work on cancer cells. And unlike cancer drugs, which require a catheter to reach the bladder, it's easy to get AITC simply by eating the right foods.

Pick the right powder. Powdered mustard, the same kind you find on the spice aisle of your supermarket, is an excellent source of this potent compound. It's made from finely ground mustard seed.

Some brands pack more than others. Researchers tested four varieties available in stores and discovered that hot, Asian mustard seed powder packed the most AITC.

Put it to work. Next, they tested it against bladder cancer cells in the lab. The Asian mustard powder:

- stopped cancer cells from multiplying.
- triggered them to self-destruct.
- kept cancer from invading the muscles in the bladder.
- squashed VEGF, a protein that prompts cancer to spread.

This last part is especially important. Bladder cancer generally doesn't become deadly until it moves into the muscles. Once that occurs, it becomes much harder to treat. Add it all up, and experts say this amazing spice could help prevent and even treat bladder cancer.

Fortunately, the part of mustard powder that kicks cancer stays fresh for a long time. Researchers stored their spice at room temperature for 10 months, then tested it again. It hadn't lost any of its isothiocyanates. And it doesn't take much for it to have an effect. In rats, a small dose of powder fought bladder cancer better than a large dose.

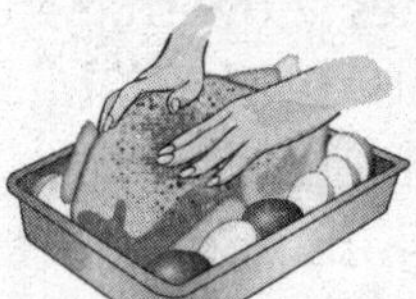

Can't-miss zesty mustard rub

1/2 cup brown sugar
4 tablespoons mustard powder
3 tablespoons black pepper
2 tablespoons chili powder
2 tablespoons ground cumin
2 tablespoons paprika
1 tablespoon garlic powder
2 teaspoons salt

Combine all ingredients in a bowl and mix thoroughly. Rub onto chicken or turkey, covering both sides. Refrigerate the poultry overnight, then cook.

Tasty treat keeps cancer at bay

Smoking, infections, arsenic in drinking water, exposure to certain chemicals, and even some drugs can cause bladder cancer, the fifth most common cancer in the United States. But eating yogurt or other fermented dairy at least twice a day could tip the odds in your favor.

Women who ate these foods were about half as likely to develop this deadly disease as women who never ate fermented dairy products. Men reaped a similar benefit, dropping their risk by more than one-third.

Fermented dairy foods boast live bacteria cultures such as *Lactobacillus casei*. These cultures protect your urinary tract from genetic changes caused by the foods you eat, changes that could lead to cancer. Foods made with fermented milk have blocked the development of bladder cancer in animal studies, too.

One particular dairy bacterium, the *Lactobacillus casei* strain Shirota, helped keep bladder cancer from coming back in people who had undergone surgery to remove cancerous tissue.

Breast cancer

Spice up your menu with this savory cancer foe

You've probably heard of turmeric. It's a bright yellow spice used in curries, soups, stews, and marinades. You might want to try it — along with adding flavor, turmeric may offer protection against breast cancer.

Prevents cancer cells from forming. A study from the University of Michigan suggests turmeric may keep breast cancer cells from multiplying. Here's how it works.

The breast contains stem cells that turn into breast cells during adolescence and breast-feeding. At other times, breast stem cells can replace old breast cells that die. But fewer new breast cells are needed in middle-aged and older adults, so limiting stem-cell growth is important. Some experts believe breast cancer starts when breast stem cells go haywire and trigger the production of cancer cells. If that's true, fewer stem cells may mean less danger of breast cancer.

Fortunately, this study discovered that stem cells treated with curcumin — the active ingredient in turmeric — made far fewer new stem cells. Normal breast cells were unaffected by curcumin. More research is needed, but this may mean turmeric could be a safe way to help prevent breast cancer without harming normal cells.

> To help your body absorb more curcumin from turmeric, flavor dishes with both turmeric and black pepper.

Reduces risk from HRT. If you use hormone replacement therapy (HRT) that combines estrogen and progestin, you may have a higher risk of breast cancer than women who use estrogen-only HRT or no HRT, studies suggest. Experts suspect progestin may

Did you know?

Wouldn't it be great if there were a single spice you could eat to help prevent cancers all over your body? Amazingly, there is. Curcumin, a natural compound found in turmeric, doesn't only fight breast cancer. It may help prevent other cancers, too.

- An Irish study found that esophagus cancer cells in a test tube died after exposure to curcumin.
- Canadian researchers killed colon cancer cells in a test tube by treating them with curcumin. And a study on animals suggests high amounts of curcumin may kill colon cancer cells.
- Lab studies have found that curcumin may trigger automatic death in leukemia cells.

Studies like these often use far more curcumin than you get from turmeric in food. Still, a few studies suggest populations that eat the most turmeric may have less risk of colon cancer and leukemia. Talk to your doctor before trying supplements because they're not safe for everyone.

increase production of vascular endothelial growth factor (VEGF), which may help breast cancer develop.

But a study found that animals given progestin and curcumin were less likely to develop breast cancer, took longer to develop tumors, and developed fewer tumors. What's more, the curcumin helped lower the production of VEGF. Scientists suspect this may be one reason curcumin made a difference.

Researchers say that you may benefit by using turmeric in your cooking. Add up to a teaspoon of this spice to casseroles, potato dishes, soups, chili, stews, curry, or tomato sauces. You can also add extra flavor to your mayonnaise, relish, or salad dressing by stirring some right into the container. Looking to spice up your egg salad? Mix in a bit of turmeric.

Pop open a pomegranate for yummy prevention

The pomegranate is not as famous as the apple, but this fruit may still help keep the doctor away. Not only does it contain health-defending antioxidants, some research suggests that munching on these tasty snacks may help slash your risk of developing breast cancer.

A laboratory study tested 10 compounds your body makes from pomegranates. These compounds are called ellagitannins, and they include ellagic acid and urolithin B. The study found that all 10 compounds could help prevent breast cancer cells from multiplying, but urolithin B was the most effective.

The researchers also discovered that six of the compounds could block the action of an enzyme called aromatase. This enzyme converts compounds called androgens into estrogen, raising the amount of estrogen in your body. That's bad because estrogen

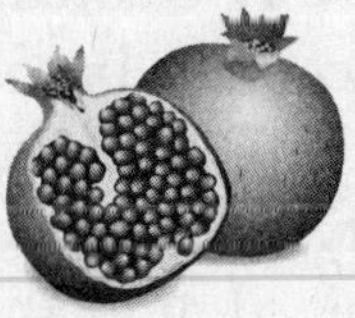

Eating a pomegranate is like opening a cereal box to get the prize inside. You don't eat the entire fruit, just the yummy juice-filled seeds. Removing the seeds can be messy and complicated — but it will not be if you try this no-fuss, no-muss method.

- Cut off the top of the pomegranate. Score the pomegranate's skin from top to bottom — without cutting into the seeds — so you can break it into one-quarter sections.
- Place the whole pomegranate in a bowl of water, break it into sections with your fingers, and roll the seeds out of each section. The seeds should sink to the bottom while the pulp around the seeds floats to the top.
- Scoop out the pulp and peel, and use a strainer to separate the seeds from the water.
- Eat and enjoy the juicy seeds.

helps breast cancer cells multiply and causes tumors to grow. In fact, some breast cancer survivors take aromatase-blocking drugs to help prevent future tumors.

Urolithin B did a better job of blocking aromatase than the other compounds, but it is still not as strong as prescription drugs. Plus it may be difficult to eat enough pomegranates or drink enough juice to get the high level of pomegranate compounds used in the study. But the researchers and other experts still believe that adding pomegranates to your diet may be a smart way to help prevent breast cancer.

Try parsnips for added protection

Bring new life to a tired old mashed potatoes recipe. Boil some parsnips, and mash them right along with the potatoes. Not only will you discover a unique new flavor in your mashed potatoes, you'll also help your body defend itself against breast cancer.

The ivory-colored, carrot-shaped parsnip may not look like a cancer defender, but it has plenty of fiber, and research reveals just how important that fiber may be. Scientists from Soochow University in China compiled the results of breast cancer studies that examined more than 700,000 women. The research revealed that the more fiber the women in the studies ate, the less likely they were to develop breast cancer. In fact, you could lower your odds by 7 percent just by eating 10 more grams of fiber every day.

Experts think fiber may help by sweeping estrogen out through your colon, which keeps it from building up in your body. Estrogen is the fuel breast tumors use to grow, so the more estrogen you have the higher your risk of breast cancer.

To add more fiber to your diet, make parsnips a regular part of your menu. One-half cup of this root vegetable contains about 3 grams of fiber. Starting with small amounts and increasing fiber gradually is a good way to avoid side effects like gas and bloating.

Choose short, fat parsnips with very little pitting. Their faintly sweet taste has hints of honey, cardamom, and butterscotch, so they are ideal for adding a new twist to soups and stews. To add even more fiber to your diet, enjoy foods like black beans, artichokes, pinto beans, raspberries, navy beans, blackberries, lentils, oat bran, and dried plums.

Baked parsnip fries

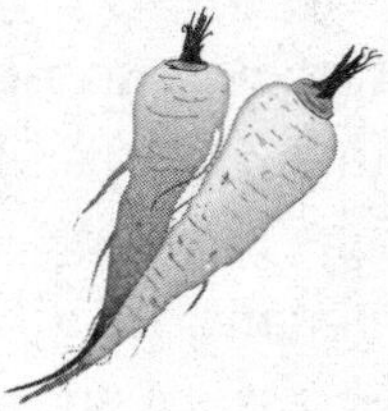

1 pound bag of parsnips

1 tablespoon olive oil

1/4 teaspoon salt

1/4 teaspoon garlic powder

Preheat the oven to 450 degrees. Wash or peel the parsnips, and cut them into french-fry style strips. Place the parsnips in a bowl, and toss with the olive oil, garlic powder, and salt. Spread the parsnips in a single layer on a rimmed baking sheet. Bake for 15 minutes, remove from the oven, and turn each parsnip with tongs or a spatula. Return to the oven, and bake for 10 to 20 minutes until the fries are golden brown. Season with ketchup, pepper, or malt vinegar, and enjoy.

Double your defense with flaxseed

Flaxseeds may be tiny, but they deliver a powerful one-two punch to help cut your breast cancer risk. Here is how they can help.

Lower your odds with lignans. Flaxseed contains compounds called lignans. A review of studies suggests that women who have passed menopause may benefit from eating foods rich in lignans. The researchers discovered that older women who ate the highest amounts of lignans lowered their risk of breast cancer. Experts are not sure why lignans help, but they have a couple of theories.

- Their high levels of antioxidants may fend off cancer.
- Lignans may limit your body's levels of aromatase, an enzyme that helps you hang on to estrogen. With less aromatase, more estrogen leaves your body during bathroom visits, so your estrogen levels sink lower. The less estrogen you have, the less likely you'll get breast cancer.

Fight back with fiber. A single tablespoon of ground flaxseed contains 2 grams of fiber. That's more fiber than a cup of raw cabbage, a raw peach, or an entire head of butterhead lettuce. Like lignans, fiber helps keep your estrogen levels low, which may further reduce your odds of breast cancer.

If you would like to try flaxseed, remember these tips.

- Grind flaxseeds with a pepper or coffee grinder before eating them. This helps your body absorb more lignans.
- Flaxseed's high fiber content makes it easy to absorb too much fiber at once, resulting in gas, bloating, and diarrhea. To prevent this, start with 1/2 teaspoon of flaxseed, and gradually work up to a tablespoon.
- Sprinkle flaxseed on hot foods such as oatmeal, or stir it into yogurt or applesauce.
- Do not use flaxseed if you have a health condition that causes diarrhea, as it may have a laxative effect. If you have a history of cancer, talk to your doctor before adding more flaxseed or eating large amounts of flaxseed.

You don't have to limit yourself to flaxseed to enjoy the benefits of lignans. Choose from a wide variety of sources including blackberries, pomegranates, buckwheat, cabbage, cranberries, garlic, kale, and broccoli.

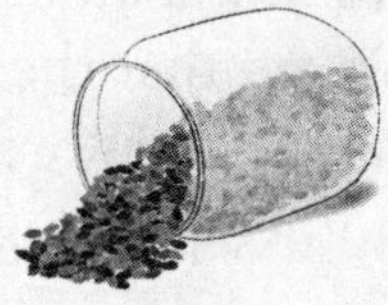

Boost the nutrition in your home recipes with this clever trick. Ground flaxseed not only contains fiber and lignans, but also alpha-linolenic acid — an omega-3 fatty acid that is good for your health. To add these nutrients to a recipe, substitute ground flaxseed for margarine, butter, or cooking oil. You can replace up to 1 tablespoon of these fats.

- Decide how much fat to replace, and multiply that amount by three. For example, to replace 1 tablespoon of margarine, you should use 3 tablespoons of ground flaxseed.
- If substituting flaxseed replaces all the fat in a recipe, add 3/4 tablespoon of liquid for each tablespoon of flaxseed you added, or add 3/4 teaspoon of liquid for each teaspoon of flaxseed added.

Just remember, baked-good recipes brown more quickly when you add flaxseed.

Enjoy the hidden cancer fighters in peaches

Juicy plums and fragrant peaches may do more than satisfy your taste buds — they may carry two concealed weapons against breast cancer.

This exciting discovery came when scientists at Texas A&M University used extracts from the "Rich Lady" peach and the "Black Splendor" plum to treat normal breast cells, cancer cells, plus cells from an aggressive type of breast cancer. Both peach and plum extracts helped keep the breast cancer cells from multiplying — even the aggressive cancer cells.

What's more, after testing several versions of the extract, they discovered that the one strong enough to kill cancer cells did not damage normal breast cells. That's good news because typical chemotherapy drugs harm both cancer cells and normal cells.

Two polyphenols in the fruits — chlorogenic acid and neochlorogenic acid — were particularly good at blocking the growth of breast cancer, and even killing cancer cells, without harming normal cells. While researchers hope to someday turn these compounds into cancer-fighting supplements, at least one expert suggests that simply eating peaches and plums may be a good way to help prevent breast cancer now.

The researchers noted that the peach extract was generally more effective than the plum extract. Enjoy raw peach slices as a snack, or try them as a topping for oatmeal, angel food cake, shortcake,

HEALTH ALERT!

A study of six peach varieties suggests at least half the chlorogenic acid in these fruits is in the peel. Unfortunately, peach peels are usually coated with more pesticides than many other fruits and vegetables. That's why experts suggest you peel your peaches before eating. To get the extra chlorogenic acid in the peel, buy organic peaches, which are pesticide-free.

If organic peaches aren't in your budget, peel the fruit. Also, try farmer's markets or buying local peaches in season. These may have fewer pesticides.

No matter what you buy, make sure you wash your peaches thoroughly under cold, running water while rubbing them clean. In fact, wash them twice. But don't use soap or detergent because they may permanently settle in the pores of the fruit.

pound cake, or even pancakes. Add peaches to a fruit salad, yogurt, or a smoothie, or use them to make jams, jellies, or yummy peach cobbler.

Sidestep cancer-causing chemicals

Barbecue, diesel exhaust, and overheated cooking oil are just three sources of cancer-causing chemicals you are probably exposed to quite often. These chemicals are called polycyclic aromatic hydrocarbons (PAHs), and they may help trigger breast cancer. Fortunately, a powerful compound found in red grapes, called resveratrol, may offer a good defense.

In researching how resveratrol fights cancer, scientists performed laboratory experiments on normal breast cells treated with a PAH. They found that applying resveratrol to these cells helped prevent cancer triggers in several ways.

- It suppressed the production of enzymes that contribute to DNA damage in breast cell genes.
- It helped reduce the PAH's ability to damage breast cell DNA.
- It helped prevent PAHs from attaching to breast cell DNA to form a "DNA adduct," a possible first step towards breast cancer.

The researchers found that breast cells were protected even when they were treated with resveratrol six hours before being exposed to the PAH. So if you're barbecuing or using cooking oil, eating resveratrol-rich foods either before or during could help protect you from these cancer-triggering chemicals.

But it wouldn't hurt to eat them on a regular basis, either. Red grapes are a good choice as they are high in resveratrol. Enjoy them as a snack, add them to fruit salad, or drink red grape juice. Other resveratrol-rich foods include dark chocolate, cocoa powder, peanuts, berries, and red wine.

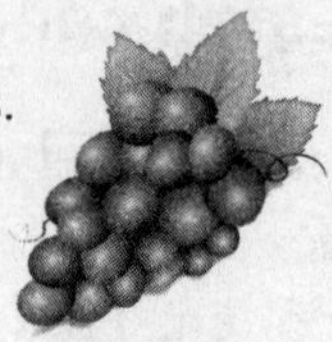

Grapes are not just for jams, jellies, and snacks. Try these clever ideas for red seedless grapes.

- Use them in place of berries in pies and tarts.
- Dip them in dark chocolate. You will end up with a lovely, sophisticated dessert that gives you even more resveratrol.
- Fit grapes into sandwiches and wraps by slicing them in half. Try them in your next chicken salad sandwich — you will be amazed at how much better it tastes.
- Substitute grapes for tomatoes in salsa and salads.
- Throw grapes in the blender whenever you make a smoothie. Leave the skins on.
- Add grapes to curry recipes.
- Include them in a fruit and cheese plate.
- For a summer treat, fill popsicle molds halfway full with grapes, and add grape juice or another favorite juice until the mold is nearly full. Freeze and enjoy.

Colds & flu

Fight back with feel-good foods

Want to avoid colds, flu, and other "bugs" this year? Don't miss the list of powerful foods that should be in your kitchen.

Yogurt. A yummy yogurt with probiotics could be just what the doctor ordered. According to a Japanese study, people who ate a small yogurt containing the probiotic *Lactobacillus bulgaricus* were less likely to catch a cold than people who drank milk instead. They also had higher natural killer cell activity.

That's good news because natural killer cells are one of your immune system's important early responders, and they may help you fend off an illness. But *Lactobacillus bulgaricus* isn't the only probiotic that can help. Studies suggest other probiotics may also help you avoid colds and other upper respiratory tract infections.

To try probiotics yourself, choose a low-fat or nonfat yogurt that contains a *Lactobacillus* or *Bifidobacterium* probiotic. They are usually labeled with an "L" such as *L. rhamnosus*, or "B" such as *B. lactis*. Also, make sure the label promises "live and active cultures," and avoid yogurts that have been heat-treated.

Apples, lentils, berries, and more. Research from the University of Illinois showed that mice that ate soluble fiber every day became less sick after infection and recovered faster than mice that ate insoluble fiber. Soluble fiber is the kind that dissolves in water. It also makes your body produce more interleukin-4 (IL-4), a protein that revs up your body's T cells to help fend off infections.

If you'd like to add more soluble fiber to your diet, start with one small serving a day and gradually add more. That can help prevent gas and other side effects. So can drinking extra water. You can find soluble fiber in apples, berries, citrus fruits, carrots, lentils, nuts, seeds, oat bran, and barley.

Green, black, or oolong tea. Children who drank 1 to 5 cups of green tea each day were less likely to get the flu, a study reported in *The Journal of Nutrition*. While that doesn't necessarily mean that adults will get the same protection, other research suggests green, oolong, and black tea have immune boosting powers.

Harvard researchers say the theanine in these teas may help boost the response of infection-fighting gamma delta T cells. These cells prompt the release of interferon, a chemical that helps you battle oncoming infections. In fact, the Harvard study found that people who drank 20 ounces of tea a day for one month produced five times more interferon than people who didn't drink tea. That may be enough to help you avoid whatever is "going around" this year.

Top-notch infection fighter

During cold and flu season, turn to garlic. It's a natural way to help your body eliminate toxins and harmful microorganisms. Eating garlic may also boost your immunity.

Experts suggest you can work up to eating as many as three cloves of garlic a day. People in China and Korea eat even more. But clear it with your doctor before adding extra garlic — especially if you take prescription medications.

If your doctor approves, start small in case you experience side effects like heartburn, gas, diarrhea, vomiting, or

> Make garlic breath vanish. Chew a few sweet-tasting fennel seeds after eating garlic to counteract the odor.

wheezing. If you tolerate garlic well, enjoy more pasta, hummus, and other garlic-laced recipes. Preserve the active ingredients in garlic by crushing the cloves, letting them sit for 10 minutes before cooking, and only cooking them lightly. If you experience problems, ask your doctor whether you can safely take supplements instead.

However it fits your lifestyle, you'll be grateful. Studies have proven that the allicin in this food kills bacteria, molds, viruses, yeasts, and parasites, making it deserving of its nickname "Russian penicillin."

HEALTH ALERT!

If you want to fight the flu, make sure you avoid drastic dieting during flu season. A Michigan State University study found that animals on a calorie-restricted diet had a higher risk of dying and took longer to recover from the flu than animals that ate normally, even though both groups ate a vitamin-fortified diet.

The researchers say calorie restriction cripples your immune system's production of natural killer (NK) cells. NK cells help control the initial rounds of the flu until your body can produce enough antibodies to fend it off. You need NK cells even if you've had a flu shot, because the shot only defends against most flu strains, not all. Your immune system must do the rest.

So forget about cutting your calories in half to lose weight during flu season. Save your dieting for the other eight months of the year.

3 things you need in your cough and cold kit

Modern scientists haven't uncovered the cure for the modern cold. But that doesn't mean you need to suffer through congestion, coughs, and other nasty symptoms.

All you need to do is stock your pantry with these three must-have ingredients. As long as you have them on hand, you'll be able to get over the virus easier and faster.

Zinc. Feel a cold coming on? The first thing you should do is reach for a zinc lozenge. Canadian researchers found that this mineral helped adults recover from a cold up to three days faster than people who didn't take zinc.

Experts say to take about 75 milligrams of zinc a day at the first sign of symptoms. But zinc supplements aren't for everyone. Some people say this mineral causes nausea and an unpleasant taste in their mouths.

Cranberries. Think cranberries only belong in your pantry during Thanksgiving? Think again. Research published in *Nutrition Journal* claims that these tart little berries are a great way to fend off cold symptoms. In a small study, people either drank a cranberry drink or a placebo for 10 weeks during cold and flu season.

The study revealed that cranberry drinkers still got sick at the same rate as people who drank the placebo. However, the cranberry group reported fewer cold and flu symptoms.

> Drop a little nutritional yeast into your soup to boost the flavor and your immune defenses. In one study during the intense months of cold season, participants who took 450 milligrams of yeast beta glucan fiber twice daily — equal to about a spoonful of nutritional yeast — for 26 weeks had significantly fewer infections than the placebo group.

Honey. Be careful if you're taking medications to counter your cold. Some cough syrups — like ones made from chlorpheniramine and hydrocodone — can kill you if you take them the wrong way. But if you have honey, you can get relief without the risks.

A review of more than a dozen clinical studies found that honey was better at reducing the severity of cough symptoms than over-the-counter medications.

Want to get even more benefits? Combine your survival kit essentials by mixing honey into a glass of cranberry juice.

Soothing honey spice tea

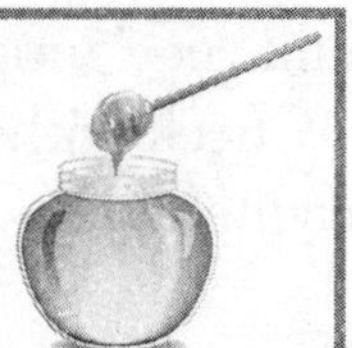

Need a sore throat cure? Try this simple but powerful tea you make from honey and three items in your spice rack. Research suggests these four ingredients have anti-inflammatory and painkilling powers.

1 clove

1/8 teaspoon powdered ginger

1/8 teaspoon powdered cinnamon

1 tablespoon honey

2 cups (16 ounces) boiling water

Mix all ingredients together, and let steep for several minutes. Sip slowly to let it soothe your throat. Drink throughout the day for the most benefit. For an extra-strength version, double the amount of ginger, and add extra honey and a few drops of lemon juice.

Boost immunity during cold season

Throw a cup of frozen peaches and a cup of frozen strawberries in a blender, add a banana and some fat-free milk, and you will have more than just a delicious smoothie. You will also have more than 300 milligrams (mg) of power-packed vitamin C in your glass. According to research, that may be a fabulous first step toward avoiding common colds this winter.

A study of more than 1,500 Swedish people found that women who took in more than 200 mg of vitamin C every day were less likely to get upper respiratory infections compared with those who got less than 100 mg a day. Men got less vitamin C from foods than women, and were more likely to benefit from taking vitamin C and vitamin E supplements.

To add more vitamin C to your diet, try these common foods that are absolutely loaded with it. Just remember that women should get 75 mg of this vitamin a day, while men should get 90 mg. Check with your doctor before drastically changing your diet or trying vitamin C supplements.

Food	Amount	Vitamin C (milligrams)
frozen peaches, sliced and sweetened	1 cup	235
raw sweet red peppers	1 cup	190
frozen mixed fruit, sweetened (peaches, cherries, raspberries, grapes, boysenberries)	1 cup	188
raw green hot chili pepper	1 pepper	109
bottled cranberry juice cocktail	8 ounces	107
frozen strawberries, sliced and sweetened	1 cup	106
boiled broccoli, drained, without salt	1 cup	101
unsweetened orange juice from concentrate	8 ounces	97
raw pineapple	1 cup	79
raw orange	1 orange	70

Herbal help to speed your recovery

You don't have time for a cold, but you're already getting that sore throat, stuffy nose, sneezing, and feeling of weakness. You probably can't avoid getting sick, but a centuries-old herbal remedy from India may make your cold shorter and milder.

Andrographis paniculata is an herb used in traditional Indian, Thai, and Chinese folk remedies. But the supplement version of this plant has been gaining popularity as a cold remedy. Several research studies explain why.

- In one study, participants who took *andrographis* showed significant improvement in coughing and nasal symptoms compared with people who took a placebo.
- Another study found that all the symptoms of people who took *andrographis* improved by the fifth day. Subjects who took a placebo reported that their coughing, headaches, or earaches didn't get any better between days 3 and 5 — and their sore throats actually got worse.
- In a Swedish study, participants who started taking *andrographis* within 36 hours of their first symptoms reported a 55 percent improvement in cough, sore throat, headache, and muscle soreness by the end of the third day.
- A systematic review of seven high-quality studies with nearly 900 participants found that *andrographis* was better than a placebo for treating the symptoms of upper respiratory tract infections like colds.

Although most studies on this herb have been supported by the manufacturer of an *andrographis* supplement, an independent review of the research found strong evidence that this herb can help treat upper respiratory tract infections like colds. Brands tested in clinical trials have included Kan Jang, ImmunoGuard, Kold Kare, and KalmCold.

If you want to try *andrographis*, keep these thoughts in mind.

- Talk to your doctor first. This herbal remedy is not safe for everyone. You may need to think twice about it if you have diabetes, take hypoglycemic drugs, or take blood-thinning drugs like warfarin (Coumadin).

- You must start taking this treatment during the first 48 hours of the cold to get good results. The correct dose varies depending on the product you choose, so follow the directions on the package.

HEALTH ALERT!

Antibacterial soaps sound attractive — why wouldn't you want to kill the bacteria on your skin? Well, they have a dirty little secret that may put your health in danger. In fact, there's a solid case for why you should never use antibacterial soap.

For starters, it isn't any more effective than regular soap. And some say that antibacterial soap may even contribute to the development of antibiotic resistant germs. Your best bet? Frequently wash your hands with plain soap. It's the surest way to avoid catching a cold.

Just scrub for a good 20 seconds — long enough to hum the "Happy Birthday" song twice. This way you'll remove germs you might otherwise transfer to your eyes, nose, and mouth, or pass on to food, surfaces, and other people.

And here's an added bonus — plain soap is typically cheaper than antibacterial varieties.

Colon cancer

Sip your way to safety

Get powerful antioxidant protection without having to eat broccoli or other vegetables. Just drink an apple smoothie, instead. Apples are chock-full of vitamins, minerals, and antioxidants known as polyphenols. These special plant compounds may account for apples' uncanny anticancer effects by:

- keeping cancerous and precancerous cells from multiplying.
- blocking enzymes that switch on cancer-causing compounds.
- triggering genes known to fight cancer.
- causing cancer cells to turn up their toes and die.

Blend up a batch of benefits. Polyphenols need to reach your colon in order to protect against colon cancer. Surprisingly, a smoothie may be the best way to get them there.

When you drink apple juice, only about one-third of its polyphenols reach the colon. The rest get absorbed by the small intestine. Nearly twice as many polyphenols reached the colon when people drank a smoothie made with 3 parts cloudy apple juice and 2 parts pureed apple, one study showed.

The pureed apples in smoothies undergo less processing than apple juice or cider. This means some of the walls surrounding apple cells are still intact. These walls seem to keep the small intestine from absorbing all the healthy, anticancer compounds. It protects them until they reach your colon.

Go whole for great protection. This study used apple smoothies made from Winesap apples. They're often used to make American cider and are jam-packed with polyphenols. Don't fret if you can't find these, though. Eating any type of apple each day can still keep the doctor away.

When comparing people with colon cancer to those without, Polish researchers found that eating an apple every day dropped the risk of colon cancer by 35 percent. Eating more than that slashed the risk in half. Apple skins pack lots of antioxidants, too, so be sure to wash the fruit and eat it whole instead of peeling it.

Maple-licious apple smoothie

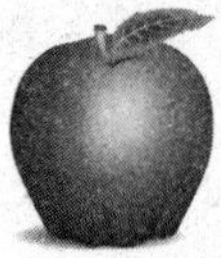

5 medium apples
1 cup cloudy apple juice
1 cup orange juice
2 tablespoons real maple syrup
1/2 teaspoon nutmeg
1/2 teaspoon cinnamon

Core and peel the apples and cut them into bite-size pieces. Place all the ingredients in a blender, adding the apple cubes first. Puree until smooth. For more antioxidants, leave the peel on the apples. For a frosty summer treat, freeze orange juice and cloudy apple juice in ice trays, then add the frozen cubes to a blender.

Veggie superstars defeat disease

Cabbage was once a "poor man's" food. Now it's a nutritional superstar. This amazingly cheap and versatile vegetable protects you against all sorts of major ailments, including colon cancer.

It's especially effective against proximal colon cancers, those that develop near the beginning of the colon. That makes sense, because tumors in the front part of the colon develop differently from those near the end.

In an Australian study, people who ate the most vegetables from the brassica family — foods like cabbage, broccoli, Brussels sprouts, and cauliflower — were a third less likely to be diagnosed with proximal colon cancer.

Brassica vegetables are loaded with glucosinolates and other plant compounds that may naturally combat cancer. They're full of folate, too, which plays a major role in keeping the genetic material in your cells healthy and normal. The bacteria in your gut break glucosinolates down into two powerful anticancer compounds.

I3C puts the crunch on cancer cells. Indole-3-carbinol (I3C) prevents cancers from forming and growing in animal studies, in part because stomach acids change it into a compound called DIM. DIM prompts the body to flush out carcinogens, or cancer-causing toxins. It also squashes inflammation, interrupts the life cycle of cancer cells, and causes them to die.

ITC sends toxins packing. Isothiocyanates (ITC) cause your body to churn out enzymes that make carcinogens harmless and help your body flush them out. Your body naturally produces these cleanup enzymes anyway, but ITC may help pump them out faster, sweeping away toxins before they do harm. ITC also keeps tumor cells from multiplying.

These same compounds may grant cabbage and its brassica cousins the ability to protect against prostate, breast, stomach, and bladder cancer, too. Plus, cabbage is high in fiber, so whether you eat it cooked or raw, it will help you stay regular.

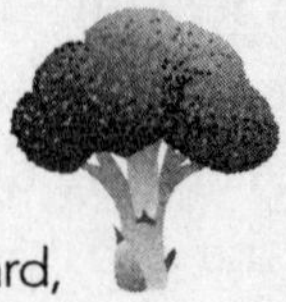

Pair broccoli with something spicy to punch up its anticancer compounds.

"Spice up your broccoli with broccoli sprouts, mustard, horseradish, or wasabi. The spicier, the better; that means it's being effective," says Elizabeth Jeffery, Professor of Nutritional Sciences at the University of Illinois.

Overcooking can sap brassicas like broccoli of their benefits. But serving them alongside a spicy condiment helps make up for the loss. Fiery foods that contain the enzyme myrosinase help broccoli produce more cancer-fighting sulforaphane. Myrosinase also helps release the anti-cancer compound earlier in the digestive process so that you absorb it sooner.

Other foods can boost broccoli's effectiveness, too. Toss in a few radish slices, a side of cabbage or Brussels sprouts, or a salad made of arugula or watercress.

Arm your defenses with a cancer-killing spice

Can you believe your kitchen cabinet contains a spice that kills cancer cells better than chemotherapy drugs? Surprising but true — as long as you have ground ginger in your spice rack.

Ginger fights inflammation, and this anti-inflammatory ability makes it effective against certain types of cancer, including ovarian and colon cancers.

Ovarian cancer strikes some 20,000 women in the United States every year — but it might be no match for ginger. In lab studies at the University of Michigan, ginger powder killed ovarian cancer cells. Ginger does the job in two ways:

- leading cancer cells to commit suicide, a process known as apoptosis

- encouraging cancer cells to digest or attack themselves, referred to as autophagy

Repeated chemotherapy treatments can make cancer cells resistant to apoptosis. With ginger, this doesn't happen. Ginger promotes autophagy, as well as apoptosis, making it a powerful weapon against ovarian cancer cells. In fact, in one laboratory study, ginger killed cancer cells better than chemotherapy drugs.

University of Michigan researchers found that ginger may also guard against colon cancer. Again, ginger's anti-inflammatory powers get the credit.

In the study, 30 people received either 2 grams of ginger supplements or a placebo each day. That amount of ginger would equal about 2 tablespoons of ground ginger. Tissue samples from the colon were also taken before and after the 28-day study.

After four weeks, samples from the people in the ginger group showed significantly lower levels of eicosanoids, inflammatory chemicals that may play a role in the development of colon cancer. Because experts think chronic inflammation in the gut may be a precursor to colon cancer, it stands to reason that ginger could offer up some potent protection against this disease.

More research is needed, but this promising study provides hope for those at risk for colon cancer. While it may be tough to get as much ginger into your diet as the people in the study, it's worth boosting your intake. People in India, China, and Japan eat lots of ginger — and these countries have lower rates of colon cancer.

You can find ground ginger in the spice aisle of your grocery store. Also look for fresh ginger root in the produce section. Both forms of ginger add flavor to foods like stir-fries, marinades, stews, sauces, or salads. Plus, you'll get a tasty dose of cancer prevention.

Savory cinnamon could save you from cancer

What if sprinkling a powder on your food every day could keep you from getting cancer? It may sound like a scam, but scientists think cinnamon may hold the key to preventing some cancers.

Cancer cells outsmart the body. Tumors need a steady blood supply in order to grow and spread. So they trick healthy blood vessels nearby. The tumor cells send out a chemical known as VEGF. It attaches to the blood vessel cells and tells them, "Hey, over here." Blood vessels then begin to grow in the tumor, giving cancerous cells the nutrients they need.

At least three hot drugs target VEGF. Experts think if they can turn off this chemical, they can starve cancer cells to death and keep them from metastasizing, or spreading to other areas. However, these drugs can have dangerous side effects, including high blood pressure, bleeding, and tears in the digestive tract.

Cinnamon puts a stop to it. Foods that naturally block VEGF could help prevent and even treat cancer. Natural compounds in cinnamon, called procyanidins, are excellent at doing just that. In fact, cinnamon packs more procyanidins than any other common food. In lab studies, these compounds shut down the activity of VEGF. Compounds in green tea, grape seeds, berries, and pomegranates have also blocked VEGF in past studies.

Cancerous tumors can lie dormant for years before you or your doctor know they're there. So foods that could stop tumors from growing and spreading are a big deal. It's not clear that eating cinnamon will have the same effect in your body that cinnamon compounds do in a test tube, but flavoring your food with it won't hurt. This study used Ceylon cinnamon *(Cinnamomum zeylanicum)* or "true cinnamon," rather than Chinese or Saigon cinnamon *(Cinnamomum cassia)*.

Surprising food packs a punch

Buckwheat is no ordinary grain. In fact, it's not a grain at all. It is the seed, or fruit, of a plant related to rhubarb. It's also tops in the mineral magnesium. One cup of buckwheat flour packs more magnesium — 301 milligrams (mg) — than a serving of nearly any other food. Buckwheat groats are no slouches either, with 86 mg per cup.

All that magnesium makes it a natural knockout against cancer. Out of 40,000 men, those who got the most magnesium in a Japanese study were least likely to develop colon cancer. Men who ate at least 327 milligrams (mg) of magnesium in their diet each day were half as likely to have colon cancer eight years later as those who got only 238 mg of this mineral. Three other studies found similar results.

Magnesium plays a major role in building and repairing DNA, the genetic material inside cells. A magnesium shortage leaves cells vulnerable to damage from oxidative stress, one cause of cancer.

- Getting enough of this mineral is even more important if you are overweight or have type 2 diabetes. Magnesium can help improve your insulin sensitivity, which in turn may help prevent colon cancer.
- Men who regularly drink alcohol reap big benefits from magnesium, too. It may offset some of the DNA damage and oxidative stress that alcohol inflicts on your cells.

Besides bolstering your body against cancer, buckwheat is naturally gluten-free. Try substituting buckwheat groats for barley or rice. Be sure to rinse them under running water first. Then add 1 cup of buckwheat groats to 2 cups of boiling water. Let the water return to a boil, reduce the heat to a simmer, cover, and cook for 15 minutes or until tender.

HEALTH ALERT!

Fruit may guard against colon cancer, but fruit juice raises your risk for rectal cancer. In one study, people who drank the most fruit juice were 74 percent more likely to develop rectal cancer than those who drank the least.

Juice contains some of the same phytochemicals as fruit but none of the fiber. And it's usually packed with added sugar. Low fiber and high sugar seem to cancel out the cancer-fighting potential of phytochemicals. Studies link high sugar, in particular, to precancerous changes in the colon.

Beat the odds with this everyday brew

There's nothing average about this Joe. Your morning cup of wake-up can tip the odds on colon cancer in your favor. A review of 24 studies revealed that:

- for every cup of coffee you drink each day, you shave your risk of colon cancer by 6 percent.
- coffee drinkers are 17 percent less likely to develop colon cancer than those who never or only occasionally drink it.
- people who drink the most java are 30 percent less likely to get this disease than those who drink the least.
- smokers and people who drink alcohol may benefit the most from coffee's protection.

Not bad for a beverage you probably drink every day. Here's a look at how it works.

Disarms cancer-causing compounds. Coffee boasts several antioxidants that block cancer and protect cells against mutation. Two in particular — cafestol and kahweol — render some carcinogens harmless. That's why it may help protect smokers. Smoking produces lots of cancer-causing compounds in your body, which coffee helps squash.

Keeps bile under control. This beverage also offsets some of the damage bile does to your colon. Bile helps break down fat from your food. If you eat a high-fat diet, you'll end up with more bile acids in your gut, which could contribute to colon cancer. An antioxidant in coffee called chlorogenic acid may protect your colon from the tumor-producing, long-term effects of bile.

Naturally fights diabetes. You're more likely to get colon cancer if you also have diabetes. The protein C-peptide is a good marker of how much insulin is in your blood. High levels of C-peptide mean your pancreas is working overtime churning out insulin — and that's not good.

One study found that women who drank more than 4 cups of coffee daily had lower levels of C-peptide. Experts think chlorogenic acid blocks your body from absorbing some of the sugar in food. That, in turn, can help prevent both diabetes and colon cancer.

Medium roast coffee contains more antioxidants than dark roast. Still, you'll lose some of these protective compounds by using paper filters. Drip-filtered coffee contains almost no cafestol or kahweol, because they get caught in the paper filter. Boiled and French-pressed coffees are much better sources of these anticancer compounds.

Unfiltered coffee can raise your cholesterol, but the same parts of the brew that boost cholesterol also contain antioxidants. Talk to your doctor about the pros and cons of unfiltered coffee if you're worried about your cholesterol.

Reel in real protection

You know fish is good for your heart, but did you know it can help prevent colon polyps, too? The omega-3 fatty acids in fish help curb inflammation that sets the stage for colon cancer. Other fats break down into compounds that cause inflammation. One of these, prostaglandin, plays a role in the formation of tumors in the intestines. The higher your prostaglandin levels, the more tumors form and the larger they grow.

That's where fish fats come in. Omega-3 fatty acids from fish may cap the production of prostaglandins in your body. Researchers wanted to see if eating fish really could help prevent polyps and, therefore, colon cancer down the road. So they asked 5,300 people what foods they ate each day. Each person also had a colonoscopy to look for polyps and cancer.

Sure enough, fish fats seemed to protect some people. Women who ate an average of three servings of fish each week were one-third less likely to have adenomatous polyps, the type most likely to turn cancerous, than women who ate only half a serving weekly. These fish lovers also got more omega-3s in their diet and had fewer prostaglandins. Although this study didn't see a benefit for men who ate the most fish, other studies have.

Not all fish are made equal, however. Some pack more omega-3 than others. Your best bets are fatty fish such as these.

- Atlantic and chinook salmon
- Atlantic and chub mackerel
- herring
- lake trout
- bluefin tuna

Some fish contain high levels of mercury and the chemical PCB. Learn how to dodge these dangers by reading "4 things you should know before eating fish" in the *Rheumatoid arthritis* chapter.

Constipation

Quick, good-tasting relief for constipation

The Greeks have known it for years, but now the secret is out. Fast relief from constipation could be hiding in your kitchen cupboard. Old-fashioned honey may be all you need to get your bowels moving.

Honey contains three types of sugar — glucose, fructose, and sucrose. Natural honeys pack more fructose than glucose. Experts think that imbalance can help loosen stool.

In most people, the small intestine can't completely absorb fructose. The result is a little like what happens when people who are lactose-intolerant drink milk. The excess fructose causes the small intestine to hold more water and sends food through the digestive tract faster.

A single dose should do the trick. Start by mixing 1 1/2 tablespoons of honey in a glass of water, the usual dose for treating constipation in Greece. This small amount had a laxative effect in one study. Wait at least 10 hours. If it hasn't helped, you can increase the dose to 3 tablespoons.

Honey may not work for everyone, but it could help some. Out of 20 people, three responded to the smaller dose, while six responded to the larger dose. You may want to avoid this home remedy if you have irritable bowel syndrome, though. The extra fructose could trigger your symptoms or make them worse.

Dried fruit fights irregularity

There's one time when fresh isn't best — when you're constipated. That's when you need the concentrated power of dried fruit.

Slash your risk of deadly diseases

Fiber may be the next super nutrient, warding off everything from stroke to pneumonia. Check out the protection you could get, just by upping your intake.

- Heart disease. Fiber improves cholesterol, insulin resistance, and blood pressure, all of which contribute to this illness.
- Hemorrhagic stroke. Overweight women who replace sugar and refined carbohydrates with high-fiber, whole-grain carbohydrates are less likely to have one.
- Type 2 diabetes. Fiber improves insulin resistance and blocks big spikes in your blood sugar.
- Colon cancer. Eating 24 grams of fiber each day may cut your risk by one-third.
- Breast cancer. Fiber may reduce estrogen in your bloodstream, a hormone that can fuel breast cancer.
- Respiratory problems such as pneumonia and flu. Fiber helps squash inflammation, which tends to worsen these diseases.
- Infectious diseases such as tuberculosis. You can once again thank fiber's impact on inflammation.

Fiber works like a chimney brush for your bowels, sweeping your system clean. Fresh fruits are good sources, but they don't pack as much fiber ounce-for-ounce as their dried counterparts. Take apples. A cup of dried apple boasts 7.5 grams (g) of fiber, more than twice as much as 1 cup of fresh apple, which contains only 3 grams.

Foods contain two types of fiber, soluble and insoluble. Experts used to think insoluble fiber worked best for treating constipation. Now they're discovering that soluble fiber acts as a laxative, too.

- Insoluble fiber bulks up stool and helps move it through the gut faster.

- Soluble fiber adds water to stool and helps it pass more easily.

Research suggests that the best foods for regular bowel movements contain a balance of both types of roughage. The two work together to pull water into stool, so it's easier to pass, and to speed up its movement through the intestines.

Researchers had 23 healthy people double their fiber intake by feeding them high-fiber cereals. Some weeks they ate cereals that contained mostly insoluble fiber in the form of bran, wheat, and corn. Some weeks they ate cereals that contained a mixture of both insoluble bran and soluble psyllium fiber. All had a positive impact on bowel movements, but the combination cereal worked best.

Dried fruits promise a good balance of both types. Five dried apricot halves, for instance, contain 1 gram of soluble and 1 g of insoluble fiber. Three dried plums provide the same.

Dietary guidelines call for adults to eat 14 grams of fiber for every 1,000 calories they eat each day. Most people only get half of that. Get a head start on your goal by checking out this list of dried super fruits that can fix constipation and get you moving again.

Dried fruit	Fiber (grams)
figs, 1 cup	14.6
pear halves, 1 cup	13.5
peach halves, 1 cup	13.1
plums, 1 cup	12.4
bananas, 1 cup	9.9
currants, 1 cup	9.8
apricot halves, 1 cup	9.5
apple slices, 1 cup	7.5
Japanese persimmon, 1 fruit	4.9

You may be worried about beefing up your fiber intake because of gas or bloating. If you add fiber to your diet gradually, you can dodge the less pleasant side effects. Drink plenty of fluids when you increase your fiber intake. Your body needs extra water to process it.

Relieve constipation with rye bread

Constipated? Give rye a try. In a Finnish study, rye bread relieved mild constipation more effectively than wheat bread or commercial laxatives.

Most people experience constipation at some point. But up to 27 percent of people in Western countries suffer from chronic constipation. That means living with symptoms like infrequent bowel movements, hard stools, and straining on the toilet. You may also experience cramps and severe stomach pain.

This study suggests that eating more rye bread can help. People in the study who ate at least 240 grams, or about six slices, of rye bread each day had an average of 1.4 more bowel movements a week. They also had softer stools and an easier time passing them.

Total intestinal transit time, which measures how long it takes for something to pass completely through the digestive tract, was also faster. Compared to people who ate wheat bread, those who ate rye bread reduced transit time by 23 percent. Compared to those taking laxatives, the rye bread group reduced transit time by 41 percent.

What makes rye bread so effective? The key is to choose whole-grain, high-fiber rye bread. Boosting your fiber intake generally improves your digestive health, but the specific types of fiber found in rye bread could play an important role in battling constipation.

Arabinoxylan, one of these important fibers, becomes fermented in the colon to form colonic short-chain fatty acids (SCFA). These SCFA may trigger contractions that speed stool through the colon and relieve constipation.

As a bonus, increased SCFA and faster transit times help lower fecal pH. That's good because a slightly acidic environment helps thwart

Did you know?

Bubbly water may be the key to getting your bowels moving. Two separate studies show that sparkling water can help ease constipation. Seniors in one study had bowel movements more often when they drank carbonated water instead of tap water. Another study found that, compared to tap water, drinking 1.5 liters — about 6 cups — of carbonated water a day eased both indigestion and constipation.

If you have these two conditions, it could be because your body moves food too slowly through your digestive tract. Sparkling water may stimulate the smooth muscles in your intestines to move things along faster. It's chock-full of minerals, too, some of which may improve constipation.

harmful bacterial enzymes, which thrive in neutral or slightly alkaline pH environments. So rye not only fights constipation — it also improves the overall health of your gut.

Adding extra fiber to your diet can sometimes cause unpleasant side effects, such as bloating or flatulence. However, the people who ate rye bread during the three-week study did not report a significant increase in these symptoms, despite an average daily intake of more than 40 grams of fiber.

If you're struggling with constipation, getting more rye bread into your diet shouldn't be too hard. Have rye toast for breakfast and make a sandwich using rye bread for lunch. Just make sure the bread is whole-grain and rich in fiber.

Surprise — milk may cure constipation

Drinking whole milk may make you constipated, but skim milk could help you get regular again. So says a small study that treated constipation with fat-free milk.

People suffering from:

- mild constipation drank 13.5 ounces of fat-free milk daily.
- moderate constipation drank 20 ounces daily.
- severe constipation drank the most, 27 ounces a day.

Meanwhile, a group of healthy volunteers tested the effects of whole milk, drinking 13.5 ounces a day for three days. The results were telling.

Skim milk stimulates bowels. The fat-free milk drinkers saw remarkable improvement. Their constipation got better, with people having more bowel movements and softer stool. Skim milk upped the levels of ghrelin and motilin in people's bodies. These two hormones stimulate your intestines to move food along. That's important, because you generally get constipated when the muscles in your digestive tract don't contract fast enough, so that stool moves through the colon too slowly.

High-fat milk hardens stool. Those drinking whole milk, on the other hand, developed harder stools. Sometimes your body doesn't absorb all the fat from food, leaving some behind in the intestines. These leftover fats, particularly saturated fat, cause stools to harden. And whole milk is high in saturated fat.

Heating milk forms natural laxative. Experts point to one more reason skim milk in this study worked as a laxative. They used UHT milk — milk that has been pasteurized using an "ultra-high temperature" technique. This special treatment turns some of the lactose in milk into lactulose, one of the most common and gentle laxatives used to treat constipation.

So look for UHT-treated milk at your local grocery. You don't have to drink your milk all at once. Break it into three smaller servings to sip during meals. Does milk give you a stomachache, bloating, or gas? Try warming it up before drinking it.

Depression

Brew more benefits from your coffee

Get ready to rev up your brainpower and mood. The caffeine in your morning cup of coffee does more than just improve your alertness and help you concentrate. Studies suggest it also boosts your short-term memory, the kind you need to temporarily remember things like directions. Caffeinated coffee can even improve your sense of well-being during the hours after you drink it. But that java can also have a far more lasting effect — it may help slash your risk of depression.

Researchers examined the coffee habits of 50,000 women and found that those who drank 2 or 3 cups of caffeinated coffee every day were 15 percent less likely to develop depression than those who drank less than a cup per week. Women who drank 4 cups daily cut their risk by 20 percent. Neither decaffeinated coffee or caffeine from other sources affected depression risk.

The researchers are not sure why the caffeine in coffee is so effective, but they point out that caffeine affects brain chemicals like serotonin, the "feel-good" neurotransmitter. They are also not sure if coffee's caffeine is the real cause behind the study results, so more research is needed.

If you don't already drink coffee, mental health experts don't necessarily encourage you to start. A sudden increase in caffeine may lead to an upset stomach, rapid heartbeat, trouble sleeping, and nervous caffeine jitters. If you are already experiencing signs of depression — loss of interest in life, deep sadness, hopelessness, or anxiety, or thoughts about suicide — skip the coffee and get professional help.

But if you have no symptoms of depression, and you already drink coffee, scientists say 2 to 4 cups daily should be safe for most adults. Just keep in mind that the researchers defined a cup of coffee as an 8-ounce beverage containing 137 milligrams of caffeine. If your brand of coffee has more caffeine or your mug is larger, you may need to adjust your servings.

To find out how much caffeine is in your coffee, check the label on the bag or can, visit the company website, or ask the barista who served you.

Did you know?

Europeans have long used St. John's wort *(Hypericum perforatum)* to fight depression without the use of drugs. Research has shown that standardized extracts of this wonder herb are effective for mild or moderate depression when taken for three months or less. At 300 milligrams two to three times a day, this natural Prozac may have fewer side effects than most antidepressants.

But it can still have negative effects, and it interacts with a wide range of drugs. So talk with your doctor before you try St. John's wort. If she gives you the green light, be patient. You may need to take this remedy for up to six weeks before you feel the benefits.

Stay sunny side up with Mediterranean food

The Mediterranean diet is not just for people with heart problems. Like heart disease, depression can affect the lining of your blood vessels and the levels of inflammation in your body. These similarities led Spanish researchers to investigate whether the heart-healthy Mediterranean diet could also help prevent depression. To start, they defined the Mediterranean diet as a food plan with these characteristics:

- high intake of fruits, nuts, vegetables, legumes, fish, and whole grains
- high amounts of monounsaturated fats like nuts or olive oil, and low intakes of saturated fat
- moderate intake of milk and dairy products
- moderate amounts of alcohol
- low intake of meat and meat products

Diet cuts depression risk. Armed with a 136-item food questionnaire, the Spanish researchers examined the diets of more than 10,000 people and rated how closely each person's diet matched the Mediterranean diet. Once they took stock of all that information, the researchers tracked the study participants' health for at least four years.

They discovered that the people who stuck the most closely to the Mediterranean diet cut their risk of depression by 30 percent. In particular, the more legumes, nuts, and fruits people ate, and the higher their ratio of monounsaturated fats over saturated fats, the more their depression risk dropped. But the more meat and dairy they ate, the more their risk rose.

Two problems need fixing. The researchers are not sure why the Mediterranean diet may fight depression. But experts suspect two things may cause depression to develop — changes in cell activities in your brain's blood vessel walls and an increase in inflammation-causing compounds called cytokines.

The cells in blood vessel walls produce a critical nerve chemical called brain-derived neurotropic factor (BDNF). Experts worry that problems with vessel walls may limit BDNF production. At the same time, eating foods high in saturated fats may help boost your cytokines. Those extra cytokines may further restrict the amount of BDNF you can make.

Less BDNF may cripple your brain's ability to protect itself against depression. Scientists have found that people with depression often have low levels of BDNF, but antidepressants help raise those levels. The Mediterranean diet acts in a similar way to lower cytokine levels and help your blood vessel walls function normally. That, in turn, may positively affect your BDNF and your brain's ability to fend off depression.

Nutrients are key players. Individual parts of the Mediterranean diet may also play special roles in preventing depression.

- Omega-3 fatty acids in fish may help fight depression and reduce the inflammatory cytokines in your body.
- Olive oil increases the activity of enzymes that help keep your brain cells healthy.
- Folic acid, B6, and B12 are crucial to processes that affect the production of serotonin and other neurotransmitters that may have feel-good powers. Their effects on the amino acids methionine and homocysteine may also help fend off depression. The Mediterranean diet is full of foods that are good sources of these B vitamins, like chickpeas and salmon.

More research is needed to confirm that the Mediterranean diet can slash your risk of depression. But why wait? You can switch to this delicious eating plan now. Start replacing junk food and trans fats with Mediterranean-style foods, and read up on the tasty Spanish, Italian, and Greek dishes that fit this diet.

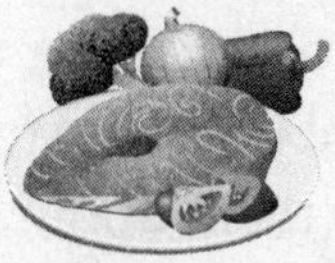

Can a salad make you happy? It might if you use these ingredients from the Mediterranean diet, topped off with a dessert of fresh fruit. These choices give you the right nutrients to help fight the blahs and avoid depression.

- spinach leaves or romaine lettuce for folic acid
- salmon for omega-3 fatty acids and vitamin B12
- chickpeas, sunflower seeds, or lentils for folic acid and vitamin B6
- chopped walnuts for omega-3 fatty acids
- sweet red peppers, tomatoes, olives, broccoli, chopped asparagus, carrots, or onion for antioxidants, monounsaturated fat, and B vitamins
- olive oil and vinegar dressing for monounsaturated fatty acids
- optional sprinkling of parmesan cheese

Lift your spirts with 5 depression busters

Want to manage your mood without turning to drugs or vitamins? Check out these lifestyle tips that will make it easier to beat the blues.

Take a stroll through nature. Start walking and you'll be healthier. But combine your walk with a nature experience — in the forest or along a lake — and the mental health benefits simply explode.

Termed walking green or walking blue, these jaunts involve nothing more than trading the traffic for the trees, the sidewalk for the sand. In studies, blue and green walkers have reported improvements in their anxiety levels, mood, and energy, compared to when they walked in the city or along a busy street.

Stay connected with supportive people. Make a point of talking to or getting together with a good friend or beloved family member. At first, aim for at least once a week. If you can, be open with them about what you're experiencing.

Break out the watercolors to lift your mood. Art therapy won't cure depression, but it can help put you on the road to recovery. That's according to a study of people with depression who took 10 hourlong sessions of art therapy as part of an overall treatment plan. Those who doodled and painted and discussed their work with an art therapist showed more improvement in their symptoms than people in a control group.

Tune in to the healing power of music. If you have the blues, try listening to the blues. Or rock, pop, jazz, or any other music you like. In a Cleveland Clinic study, people who listened to either their favorite music or soothing tunes eased their depression symptoms by 25 percent.

Give bad sleep habits a wake-up call. Find yourself cranky and grumpy after tossing and turning all night? Poor sleep is both a common symptom and a risk factor for depression.

But getting a good night's rest may help, according to a small study of people with insomnia. They received cognitive behavioral therapy, a treatment that included visits to a specialist who helped them change their sleep habits. Those who showed improvements in their sleep also reported feeling less depressed.

Diabetes

Banish diabetes with blueberries

Long after Fats Domino found his thrill on Blueberry Hill, researchers found some thrilling news about blueberries. These tiny berries may play a big role in preventing diabetes.

Here's how a simple snack food switch can help you control your blood sugar. Just whip up a blueberry smoothie instead of chomping on potato chips or other unhealthy fare.

Researchers at Louisiana State University System's Pennington Biomedical Research Center discovered that two blueberry smoothies a day helped improve insulin sensitivity in obese, insulin-resistant people — the kind of folks at high risk for type 2 diabetes.

Insulin resistance means your body produces the hormone insulin but doesn't use it properly. You need insulin to help convert glucose, a type of sugar, into energy. Cells have insulin receptors that work like locks on a door, and insulin is the key. After a meal, insulin fits into the keyhole, or receptor, and the cell opens to let in glucose from your blood.

When muscle, fat, and liver cells become insulin resistant, they stop responding properly. Insulin can't unlock them, so glucose can't enter. Sugar then begins to build up in your blood.

Eventually, this high blood sugar can lead to diabetes. Improving your insulin sensitivity, or how your body responds to insulin, can help keep your blood sugar under control.

The 32 people in the six-week study snacked on smoothies around breakfast and dinner. Some got smoothies made with freeze-dried, whole blueberries crushed into a powder. Each day, they received the equivalent of about 2 cups of fresh, whole blueberries. Others got placebo smoothies, which contained the same amount of calories but no blueberries. Keep in mind that they didn't just add smoothies to their diet. They also cut calories elsewhere, so their overall food intake remained the same.

In the blueberry group, 67 percent of the people had a 10 percent or greater improvement in insulin sensitivity, as measured by the state-of-the-art hyperinsulinemic-euglycemic clamp technique. Their average change was 22.2 percent, compared to 4.9 percent for the placebo group.

Credit goes to the high content of phytochemicals in blueberries, especially anthocyanins — powerful antioxidants that give blueberries their color. Researchers aren't sure exactly how they work their magic, but they seem to have a direct effect. That's because nothing else changed between the two groups, including body weight, inflammation, cholesterol, and blood pressure.

Besides being packed with phytochemicals, blueberries are also rich in fiber and vitamin C, making them an all-around healthy snack. Blending them into smoothies is one cool trick to sneak more of these powerhouses into your diet. You can also sprinkle some on your breakfast cereal, mix them into a fruit salad, or just eat a bowl of blueberries for dessert. However you do it, eating more blueberries can be a delicious way to defend yourself against diabetes.

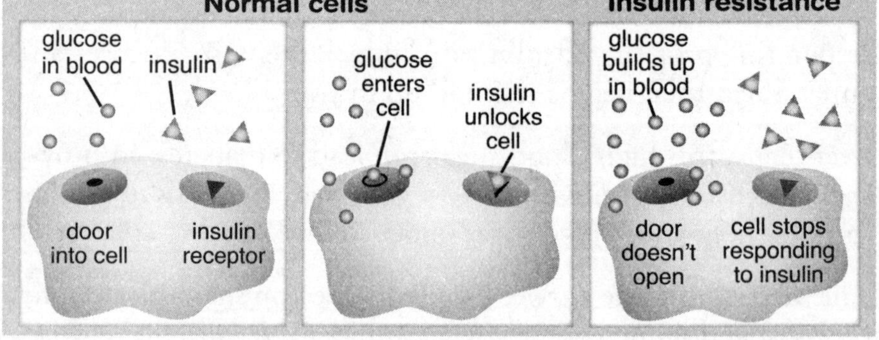

Just think — the ultimate anti-diabetes treatment may be sitting in your refrigerator right now. Now that's quite a thrill.

Sweet & fruity smoothie

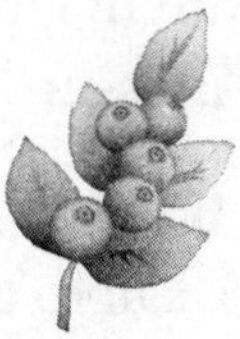

1 cup frozen blueberries
1 cup low-fat honey-vanilla Greek-style yogurt
1 cup 1-percent milk
4 to 6 ice cubes

Combine all ingredients in a blender and blend until smooth. Serve in chilled glasses and enjoy. Makes two smoothies.

Spice up the fight for lower blood sugar

Want to ward off diabetes? Then spike your meals with high-magnesium foods and spices, like sunflower seeds, navy beans, mustard, sage, and oregano.

This much-needed mineral helps your body process glucose, or sugar. Without enough magnesium inside them, cells stop responding to insulin. They become less sensitive. Unfortunately, low magnesium levels create a catch-22. Insulin has a hard time entering cells that are low in magnesium, but cells need insulin in order to stock up more of this mineral.

Research points to just how important this mineral can be in preventing blood sugar disorders. Out of nearly 5,000 people, those who got the most magnesium — whether from food or supplements — had half the risk of developing type 2 diabetes as those who routinely got the least. They also had fewer inflammation-causing compounds in their bodies. Inflammation makes your cells less sensitive to insulin.

That's just for starters. Foods full of magnesium could save you from more than diabetes.

High blood pressure. People who eat fruits and vegetables rich in the minerals magnesium and potassium consistently have lower blood pressure than other people. One study found that the more magnesium women got from food, the more their blood pressure dropped.

Weak bones. Several studies suggest this mineral improves bone density. Fail to get enough magnesium, and your body won't process calcium or regulate it properly.

Colon cancer. Fitting more magnesium into your diet could cut your risk of colon cancer. It seems to work hand in hand with calcium to stop cancer cells in the colon wall from multiplying. Together, these minerals may also prevent colon polyps from coming back.

You can boost your magnesium naturally by eating the usual suspects, like bananas and milk. But plenty of interesting spices and foods are great sources, too. Branch out with these delicious disease fighters.

Item and serving size	Magnesium content (milligrams)
navy beans, 1 cup cooked	96.5
sunflower seeds, toasted, 1/4 cup	43.3
pumpkin seeds, roasted, 1/4 cup	42.0
celery seed, 1 teaspoon	8.8
ground mustard seed, 1 teaspoon	7.4
dill seed, dried, 1 teaspoon	5.4
basil, dried leaves, 1 teaspoon	5.0
sage, ground, 1 teaspoon	3.0
oregano leaves, dried, 1 teaspoon	2.7

Coffee gives you an edge

Your coffee craving could secretly save you from diabetes. Women who drink 4 cups of coffee a day have half the chance of developing type 2 diabetes as nondrinkers. So says a study from the University of California, Los Angeles.

Scientists have been debating about the reasons behind coffee's protective power. This study adds yet another twist. Women who drank the most caffeinated coffee a day had higher levels of a protein known as SHBG. That protein plays a role in the development of type 2 diabetes — people with more SHBG are less likely to get the disease.

Decaf coffee didn't affect SHBG, so caffeine may deserve at least some credit. Caffeine isn't the only thing coffee has going for it. It's also:

- rich in magnesium, which makes your cells more sensitive to insulin.
- loaded with lignans, compounds that prevent diabetes in lab studies.
- brimming with potassium, a mineral important for secreting insulin.
- chock-full of chlorogenic acid, an antioxidant that boosts insulin sensitivity and lowers blood sugar in experiments.

In fact, this last coffee compound could explain why drinking coffee with your lunch, rather than with breakfast, may have the biggest impact on prevention. Women who drank more than 1 cup of coffee with lunch, whether regular or decaf, were one-third less likely to develop diabetes.

Chlorogenic acid can make your digestive tract absorb sugar more slowly. This keeps your blood sugar from spiking after a meal. Drinking a cup of coffee with a large meal, like lunch or dinner, could help prevent the kind of blood sugar highs that contribute to diabetes.

So go ahead, fill your cup to the brim — just drink it black. Adding milk may blunt some of its protection. Avoid regular coffee if you have diabetes, however. Caffeine may actually worsen blood sugar control in people who already have this disease. Play it safe and stick to decaf.

HEALTH ALERT!

Drinking water could be the cheapest, easiest way to ward off diabetes. Dehydration is directly linked to high blood sugar. When your body runs low on water, it sends out a distress signal in the form of vasopressin. This hormone tells your kidneys to hold on to more water.

Vasopressin affects other things, too — namely, blood sugar. It tells your liver to crank out more glucose, which raises your blood sugar. Researchers studied more than 3,000 middle-aged French adults, asking how much water they drank during the day. All had normal blood sugar at the start of the study.

After nine years, people who drank less than 17 ounces (a little more than two cups) each day were nearly one-third more likely to have diabetes than people who drank more than 34 ounces (about a quart) of water daily.

Great reason to swap brown rice for white

Harvard researchers found that eating white rice five or more times a week made people 17 percent more likely to develop diabetes. Replacing as little as 1/4 cup with brown rice reversed that trend, lowering their risk by 16 percent.

Unlike white rice, brown rice is a powerhouse of nutrition because it hasn't been processed. White rice has been milled and polished. This strips away key nutrients, including fiber. Both types contain plenty of carbohydrates, but the fiber in brown rice keeps those carbs from hitting your bloodstream all at once. Your body absorbs them more slowly than the carbs in white rice, which helps avoid big blood sugar spikes.

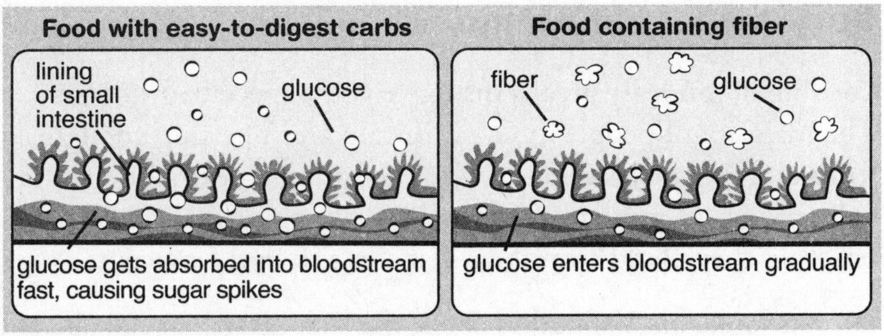

Processing also removes other nutrients that guard against diabetes, like lignans, phytoestrogens, vitamins, and minerals — including magnesium.

Can't stand brown rice? Replacing white rice with other whole grains, such as barley or whole wheat, offered similar protection in this study. Or start the day with a steaming bowl of oatmeal. Its soluble fiber offers special protection from diabetes. It slows down the movement of food from your stomach to your intestines. This means sugar enters your bloodstream gradually. But that's not all. Eating this 25-cent meal delivers huge heart benefits, too.

- lowers your blood pressure, bolstering your body against heart attack, stroke, and heart failure
- reduces your total and LDL, or "bad," cholesterol levels, protecting against heart attack and stroke
- helps manage your blood sugar, warding off heart attacks in people who have diabetes

All oatmeal is whole grain, whether it's instant, quick, or slow-cooking. Prepare your favorite type and enjoy.

Supercharge your oatmeal with a dollop of canned pumpkin. You'll get even more diabetes-fighting fiber in your diet, plus an immune-boosting shot of vitamin A. Top it off with a dash of cinnamon and handful of chopped walnuts for a perfect winter breakfast.

Go green for natural protection

Loading up on leafy greens may give you a special advantage. The majority of people in Great Britain aren't getting enough fruits and vegetables each day. But by eating an extra one-and-a-half servings of leafy green vegetables, like spinach, cabbage, or broccoli, they could trim their diabetes risk by 14 percent.

Experts looked at six studies about the link between vegetables, fruits, and diabetes. They discovered that people who ate the fewest leafy greens were more likely to develop type 2 diabetes down the road. Eating an extra one-and-a-half servings daily, however, reversed that danger.

The portions add up fast. Here's what a serving and a half looks like — after cooking — for these common greens.

spinach	2/3 cup
broccoli	3/4 cup
cabbage	3/4 cup
Brussels sprouts	6 sprouts
cauliflower	7 flowerets

Vegetables provide lots of antioxidants that safeguard your cells against the damage done by oxidative stress. Leafy green vegetables like spinach are an especially good source. They're packed with polyphenols, vitamin C, and beta carotene — all powerful antioxidants.

Plus, they're excellent sources of magnesium, a mineral linked to a lower risk of diabetes. Leafy green vegetables are also a good source of linolenic acid, an important type of polyunsaturated fat known as omega-3. This fat makes your muscle cells more sensitive to insulin. Add it all up, and you can't go wrong. So pile your plate high for better health.

HEALTH ALERT!

Selenium overload can be a secret cause of hair loss, joint pain, fatigue, and even damaged fingernails. You need this mineral in small amounts for good health, but it's easy to exceed the safe range with supplements. Skip selenium supplements unless your doctor specifically recommends them. A balanced diet with plenty of unprocessed foods should supply all you need.

Multi-talented mineral beats disease

Get just the right amount of one essential nutrient, and you'll better your chances of avoiding type 2 diabetes. It's the trace mineral selenium, and too little in your diet may make you more likely to develop diabetes.

For nine years, researchers periodically measured selenium levels in the blood of nearly 1,200 French seniors. Then they compared each person's selenium levels to their blood sugar levels. Men with the most selenium were half as likely to develop diabetes as those with the least.

This mineral is a key part of certain proteins that protect your cells from oxidation. Selenium may also make your cells more sensitive to insulin. However, men and women tend to process it differently. That likely explains why only men, not women, seemed to benefit from higher levels.

Before you run out and stock up on supplements, consider this — having too much selenium in your system could just as easily increase your risk of diabetes. It's a fine line. Taking large amounts in the long term may permanently change the way insulin works in your body. Two separate studies found that taking as little as 200 micrograms of selenium a day in the form of supplements slightly raised the type 2 diabetes risk in men, especially in men who were already getting plenty from food.

Your best bet — eat a balanced diet that includes selenium-rich foods like fish, whole grains, and lean beef. Halibut, orange roughy, and light tuna are excellent seafood sources. Meat eaters will love knowing top sirloin, bottom round, and eye of round are top-notch, too. And don't discount these good sources — ricotta cheese and couscous.

Tangy fruit stops slide toward diabetes

An everyday breakfast food could help your body use insulin more efficiently and protect your cells from damage. The compound naringin gives grapefruit and other citrus fruits their bitter flavor, but it's also a potent force in fighting diabetes.

This compound turns on a receptor in your body called PPARy, the same one targeted by prescription medicines. Here's what PPARy can do.

- It makes your cells respond better to insulin. Usually, insulin resistance causes your beta cells, the ones that make insulin, to shrink in size and eventually stop working. Naringin kept that from happening in lab rats.
- It protects muscle, liver, and beta cells from the ravages of inflammation and oxidation. In one study, the more naringin rats were given, the more protected they were from inflammation.

Chronic inflammation can cause insulin resistance throughout your body. By turning on PPARy and blocking oxidation, naringin could keep your body from pumping out inflammatory compounds.

Of course, grapefruit are great when you're watching your waistline. Your gut breaks naringin down into naringenin, which may cause your liver to burn fat instead of storing it. And at only 52 calories, you can't go wrong with half a grapefruit at breakfast. Plus, this tart and tasty delight is loaded with important vitamins, including vitamins A and C, and minerals like potassium. It's also full of soluble fiber, which helps improve digestion and control the absorption of fat in your intestines.

Unfortunately, this citrus fruit and its juice can interfere with some medications, like statin drugs. Ask your doctor or pharmacist if it's safe to make grapefruit a regular part of your diet.

Honey-marinated grapefruit

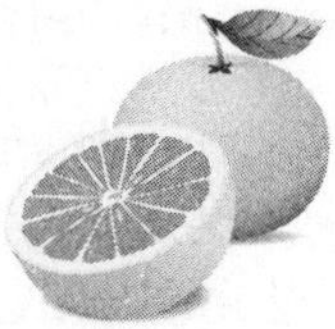

2 tablespoons honey

4 red grapefruit

Grate 1 tablespoon of rind from one grapefruit. Slice that fruit in half and squeeze the juice into a container. Peel the three remaining grapefruit, trimming away as much of the white pith as possible. Separate the sections and place them on a platter. Pierce each section with a fork. Microwave 2 tablespoons of honey in a bowl until warm. Add grapefruit juice and grated rind, and mix well. Drizzle mixture over grapefruit sections. Let stand for 15 minutes before serving so that the marinade seeps into the fruit.

Hit the produce aisle for top-notch protection

Grab a bunch of broccoli raab the next time you're in the supermarket. Put this leafy green at the top of your grocery list if you're worried about developing diabetes.

Why? It's a top source of vitamin K, and evidence suggests that people who get the most vitamin K in their diets are least likely to get diabetes. This nutrient comes in two forms — phylloquinone and menaquinones. Dutch researchers discovered that out of 38,000 people:

- those who got the most phylloquinone were 19 percent less likely to develop type 2 diabetes.

- those who got the most menaquinone were 7 percent less likely. Menaquinone seemed to boost HDL cholesterol, too, and squash inflammatory compounds in the body.

Vitamin K goes into making osteocalcin. This bone-building protein also acts like a hormone, prompting your pancreas to release more insulin and making your cells more sensitive to insulin. And by easing inflammation, vitamin K could further improve insulin sensitivity.

Fortunately, this nutrient is easy to find. Green, leafy vegetables like broccoli raab, kale, collards, and spinach are the best sources of phylloquinone. You'll find menaquinone in meat, eggs, and cheese. Eat a variety of foods for all the vitamin K you need to fight disease.

A word of caution — if you take a blood thinner like Coumadin, talk with your doctor before changing your diet. Adding vitamin K could change the way the drug works.

Hidden benefits of whole milk

Forget about low fat. Go whole if you're worried about blood sugar. Sure, you've had it drummed into your head that dairy fat is bad for you — bad for your heart, bad for your waistline, bad for diabetes. Not so, says a succession of new research and a growing chorus of experts.

Secret ingredient. Whole-fat milk, cheese, yogurt, and butter contain a fat known as trans-palmitoleate. Most studies up until now have measured how much dairy people eat each day. But a new study asked a different question — how much trans-palmitoleate do they have in their blood?

Surprising results. Researchers asked more than 3,700 people what they ate each day. Three years later, they tested their blood for trans-palmitoleate. Those who ate the most whole-fat dairy foods had the highest levels. And those with the highest levels were almost three times less likely to have diabetes 20 years later. In addition, they:

- were less resistant to insulin.
- had less body fat, despite eating plenty of dairy fat.
- had higher levels of "good" HDL cholesterol and lower triglycerides.

Add it up, and this compound could explain why people who eat lots of dairy have a lower risk of type 2 diabetes. Trans-palmitoleate may work the same way as a compound your body normally makes on its own, called cis-palmitoleate. This seems to keep the liver from churning out fats that would otherwise lead to insulin resistance. It may tell your muscle cells to pull glucose out of the bloodstream, too. However it works, cis-palmitoleate improved insulin resistance and other metabolic problems in animal studies.

However, it can't counteract the effects of all the carbohydrates and empty calories most people eat. Eating unhealthy foods overwhelms your body's natural diabetes defenses. That's where whole-fat dairy comes in. It gives you a dose of trans-palmitoleate, which picks up the slack.

Good news for you. Lots of people think dairy foods contribute to heart disease. Surprisingly, many health experts say that's not the case. Dairy foods can actually boost your good HDL cholesterol and lower your blood pressure. Experts looked at several recent studies on the link between dairy and disease. Compared to people who ate the least dairy every day, those who ate the most were:

- 8 percent less likely to get heart disease.
- 21 percent less likely to have a stroke.
- 15 percent less likely to get diabetes.
- 13 percent less likely to die from any cause.

So don't think of dairy as a dirty word. Although it contains saturated fat, research shows that dairy fat doesn't boost your risk for heart disease or diabetes. Besides, milk, cheese, and yogurt pack plenty of other nutrients. Together, they make for powerful allies against disease.

> **Did you know?**
>
> Just because a food says "no sugar" doesn't mean it won't send your blood sugar skyrocketing. Don't get taken by surprise. Foods without sugar can still be chock-full of carbohydrates. Check the listing for "Total Carbohydrate" on the Nutrition Facts label.
>
> Look at the serving size while you're at it. Otherwise, for example, you could find yourself pouring too much cereal into your bowl each morning. When that happens, you wind up consuming way more sugar, fat, and calories than you think. So be mindful of portion sizes and how much you eat. Doing so will help you avoid blood sugar spikes and prevent weight gain over time.

'Health' foods could harm more than help

A common food additive could be setting you up for diabetes. Carrageenan, made from red algae, is in everything from reduced-fat dairy (ice cream, yogurt, whipped cream, and soy milk) to diet drinks and low-fat processed meats. That's because it improves the texture of reduced-fat and other "diet" foods.

It also causes inflammation by triggering an immune response. In fact, researchers have used it for decades to cause inflammation in test-tube and animal experiments. Lab studies suggest this same inflammatory response throws off the way insulin works in your body. This, in turn, worsens insulin resistance and could contribute to type 2 diabetes.

Even more worrisome, these negative effects happened with much less carrageenan than the average person eats each day. Carrageenan has been added to more and more foods over the last 50 years in an effort to make them healthier and tastier. During that same time, diabetes has become an epidemic.

Check the ingredient list of reduced-fat and other diet foods and drinks for carrageenan. Focus on eating fresh, unprocessed foods when possible.

Eat this to avoid complications

Salmon, milk, and fortified dairy foods could prevent diabetes. For people who already have the disease, the vitamin D in these foods could save them from blindness and kidney failure.

This essential nutrient does more than build strong bones. It also helps regulate your blood sugar levels. Experts aren't certain why, but it may naturally boost your body's production of insulin.

Lots of people with diabetes have a shortage of vitamin D. They often go hand in hand. And the less vitamin D you have in your blood, the higher your blood sugar and the worse your insulin resistance tend to be. In one study, nine out of 10 people with diabetes didn't have enough vitamin D in their bloodstream. The lower their vitamin D levels, the higher their HbA1c, which occurs when hemoglobin joins with glucose in the blood. The more glucose in the blood, the more hemoglobin will be present.

Low vitamin D can wreak havoc on your heart and eyes, too. People who have diabetes and a vitamin D shortage:

- have twice the risk for heart disease and a higher risk of stroke and heart attack.

- are more likely to develop diabetic retinopathy, a leading cause of blindness.

By helping to control your blood sugar, vitamin D could help you dodge other complications, such as kidney failure. Diabetes is the top cause of kidney failure in the United States.

Eating more vitamin D-rich foods may dial back these dangers. In one study, people with type 2 diabetes drank a yogurt-based beverage fortified with 500 international units (IU) of vitamin D twice a day. This gave them a total of 1,000 IU of vitamin D each day, in addition to what they got from other foods and sunlight. Twelve weeks later, they had:

- lost weight.
- shed body fat.
- lowered their triglycerides.
- improved their insulin resistance.

Fortified dairy products, like milk, are among the best sources of vitamin D. So are fatty fish, such as salmon, mackerel, and tuna. Still, some people may need supplements — particularly older adults, obese people, and those with dark skin, all of whom are more likely to be vitamin D-deficient.

Talk to your doctor before taking supplements. Getting too much vitamin D can cause calcium to build up to dangerously high levels in your blood.

Put a lid on post-meal spikes

Eating breakfast can keep your blood sugar from jumping after lunch. But what about preventing post-breakfast spikes? Try an early-morning snack.

In a small study, 10 people with diabetes ate a high-protein, low-carbohydrate snack two hours before breakfast. Then, on a different morning, they skipped the snack and just ate breakfast. Researchers measured their blood sugar both mornings. Sure enough, their post-breakfast blood sugar was 40 percent lower the morning they ate a snack.

The key — eating something high in protein about two hours before breakfast. In this case, a high-protein snack meant 3 tablespoons of soybeans and 2.5 ounces of yogurt. Whatever you choose, enjoy it first thing in the morning. Wait a couple of hours, then sit down to your regular breakfast.

Popular drink blunts sugar spikes

Simply sipping black tea with meals could help control dangerous blood sugar spikes. This delicious beverage is packed with polysaccharides, antioxidants that may keep your blood sugar from surging after you eat.

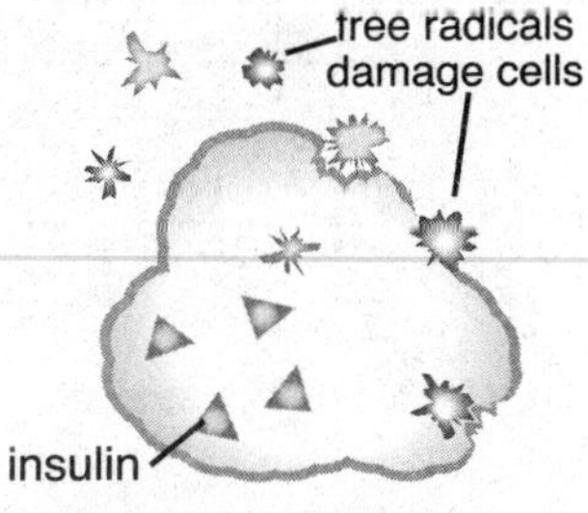

Controlling these ups and downs is crucial. Blood sugar tends to rise sharply after meals, as your small intestine absorbs the glucose from food. Unfortunately, high blood sugar — especially following a meal — creates dangerous free radical compounds. These damage cells throughout your body but wreak particular havoc on the ones that make insulin.

Over time, blood sugar spikes can damage your eyes, kidneys, nerves, and blood vessels, plus contribute to heart disease and high blood pressure.

Fend off free radicals. Polysaccharides act as antioxidants, protecting cells from free radical damage. And although green and oolong tea also contain antioxidants, black tea antioxidants were stronger in one study.

Keep sugar levels stable. A big part of diabetes management is keeping your blood sugar levels stable and avoiding ups and downs. The polysaccharides in black tea may help. Lab studies show they stop your small intestine from absorbing some of the glucose, or sugar, from food. Normally, enzymes break down carbohydrates into glucose. The black tea compounds tie up these enzymes so they can't do their job, and the carbs pass through without being absorbed.

Certain diabetes drugs aim to do the same thing. Unfortunately, medications that block carbohydrate-digesting enzymes also block the ones that break down starches. The starches then ferment in your digestive tract, with some unpleasant side effects. Unlike these drugs, drinking black tea won't cause bloating, gas, or diarrhea. So steep a hot cup and toast to your health.

A well-timed "dose" of vinegar can blunt blood-sugar spikes and keep your glucose under control. Just dress your salad with 2 tablespoons of vinegar and eat it at the start of your meal to curb blood sugar increases afterward. Vinegar slows the absorption of glucose into your bloodstream.

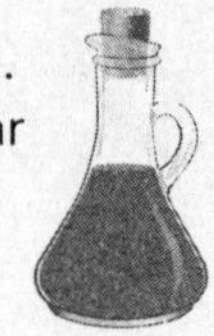

Choose carbs wisely to lower blood sugar

It's a tried-and-true strategy, and the evidence supports it — eating mostly low-GI foods can guard against diabetes and other deadly diseases.

The Glycemic Index (GI) measures a food's ability to raise your blood sugar. Some foods contain carbohydrates that get digested slowly, giving them a low GI. Other foods contain carbs that are digested quickly, making them high-GI. Carbs that break down slowly boast big advantages. Stick with them, and you could slash your risk of:

- type 2 diabetes.
- heart disease.
- macular degeneration.
- cataracts.

Here's a look at how low-GI foods impact your body.

Squash insulin resistance. Your cells naturally respond less to insulin as you age, a problem known as insulin resistance. Eating mostly high-GI foods worsens insulin resistance. That, in turn, makes you more likely to develop high blood sugar, high cholesterol, and high blood pressure — a perfect recipe for heart disease. High-GI foods also lower your "good" HDL cholesterol, raise triglycerides, and boost inflammation throughout your body. Carbs that digest slowly, on the other hand, help stop this trend.

Fight high blood sugar. Low-GI foods may still contain carbohydrates. They simply release their sugar into your bloodstream gradually, which helps prevent high blood sugar. That's important, because high blood sugar contributes to insulin resistance. Anything that keeps a lid on blood sugar also cuts your body's need for insulin, along with your risk of type 2 diabetes.

You'll reap big benefits even if you already have this disease. Eating mostly low-GI foods can improve blood sugar control, lower HbA1c, and reduce your number of hypoglycemic — or low blood sugar — episodes.

Guard organs against sugar spikes. The heart, brain, and retina rely on rapid blood flow to function. A sudden spike in blood sugar can damage these delicate organs. Because the carbs in low-GI foods break down slowly, their sugar doesn't hit important organs all at once.

Shifting to a low-GI diet doesn't have to be hard. A few smart substitutions can ease the way without making you feel deprived.

- Opt for fruits with a low GI, for instance, in lieu of those with a higher-GI. Snack on apples, pears, citrus fruits (oranges, grapefruits, tangerines), and berries (strawberries, raspberries, cranberries, blackberries, blueberries).
- Skip tropical fruits like mangoes, guava, bananas, grapes, raisins, watermelon, and cantaloupe. They have a higher GI.
- Boil, don't bake, yams, potatoes and plantains. The boiled versions tend to have a lower GI.
- Chill boiled potatoes and serve them cold.
- Add a dash of vinegar, lime, or lemon juice to carbohydrates. The acid in them slows digestion, so sugars get absorbed into your blood much more slowly.
- Parboil rice. Pressure cooking rice instead of steaming it could slash its GI by as much as 30 percent.

News about the Glycemic Index

Some foods have a surprisingly high Glycemic Index (GI). For example, whole-wheat breads can have a GI similar to breads made from white flour. Look for products that contain intact whole grains, not simply those labeled "whole wheat."

Not all foods with a low GI are healthy. Some are full of bad fats, either naturally or because manufacturers have replaced the carbohydrates with fat to lower the GI. Read the Nutrition Facts label on food to get the whole picture.

- Avoid overcooking pasta. Al dente, or slightly firm, pasta has a lower GI.

You can look up the GI of specific foods for free on websites such as *glycemicindex.com*.

Control sugar without counting

Here's an easy way to lower your blood sugar without counting carbohydrates or worrying about the Glycemic Index. Eat the vegetables on your plate before anything else.

People with diabetes who ate their vegetables first at each meal, before chowing down on carbs or meat, saw bigger drops in their HbA1c levels than people who stuck to the traditional diabetes exchange meal plan. Both groups made gains in controlling their blood sugar over two years, but the veggies-first group saw the most improvement.

A plan like this couldn't be simpler. Include vegetables with your major meals, and polish off that portion of your plate before moving on to the other food.

Sweet solution tames diabetes

One humble spice can lower cholesterol, blood sugar, and blood pressure, and even relieve inflammation in people with type 2 diabetes. It's cinnamon, and study after study adds to the proof of its healing power.

This spice may fix problems with the way insulin affects your cells.

- It seems to work similarly to the diabetes drugs thiazolidinediones, making your cells more responsive to insulin so they use it better.

- It also helps squelch inflammation throughout the body. Inflammation plays a major role in the development of diabetes complications.

Can you guess the emergency food that every person with diabetes should keep on hand? If you're thinking of candy, try again. It's glucose tablets. They're convenient, cheap, and lifesaving. Research indicates that these chewable tablets work more quickly to raise low glucose levels than sugars from food, making them the best choice.

Cinnamon lowers fasting blood sugar, but some research suggests it does more. For instance, you may have diabetes, but you don't have to have high cholesterol. Research shows cinnamon may help bring it down in people with type 2 diabetes. It may also lower your blood pressure, improve insulin sensitivity, and reduce your blood sugar after eating.

Best of all, you don't need much cinnamon to get benefits like these. People who took just 3/4 teaspoon a day in one study saw a significant drop in their HbA1c levels, from 8.22 to 7.86. Their blood pressure decreased, too.

Not every study on cinnamon has found that it helps blood sugar. But they may not have lasted long enough. It could take 12 weeks of taking the spice daily in order to see a difference. Some studies only lasted six weeks.

The type of cinnamon may also matter. Most studies used spice made from the *Cinnamomum cassia* tree, but you can buy other varieties, including *Cinnamomum zeylancium* or "true cinnamon."

Keep in mind, this spice is not a cure-all for diabetes. Take it alongside your regular diabetes medicines, however, and experts say it may give you an edge in managing the disease.

Diverticulitis

Cut meat to curb belly pain

Vegetables — and fruits and nuts and whole grains — may be just what your intestines crave. That's because people who avoid eating meat and focus instead on nonmeat foods are 30 percent less likely to develop diverticular disease, research says.

About half of Americans ages 60 to 80 have diverticulosis, or small pouches that bulge out in the intestinal wall. These weak spots may not cause any symptoms, but they can develop into infected areas, a painful condition called diverticulitis. A bout of this illness may cause pain on the lower left side of your abdomen. You may also have fever, nausea, chills, trouble with bowel movements, and difficulty urinating.

You may be able to steer clear of the common age-related condition of diverticular disease by focusing on plant rather than animal foods, as the research showed. Experts have two theories about why a vegetarian diet may help.

Fiber soothes intestines. In one study, people who ate lots of fiber — more than 25 grams (g) per day — had the lowest risk of developing diverticular disease. Eating fiber helps bulk up stool and reduce the amount of time it stays in your intestines. That seems to lead to less pressure against the intestinal walls and less chance of pouches forming.

The average American over age 50 eats about half the recommended 25-35 g of fiber per day, a far cry from the healthiest folks in the study. You can add more fiber to your diet by focusing on whole-grain breads and cereals, fresh fruits and vegetables, and beans.

Helpful bacteria protect colon wall. Your digestive tract is home to millions of bacteria, many of which help out by aiding digestion and stopping the growth of disease-causing bacteria. When you eat meat, the types of bacteria that live in your colon are different from those in the colons of vegetarians. This change might make your colon wall weaker and more prone to damage from diverticular disease.

Nutty snacks may help — not hurt

Doctors since the 1950s have told people with diverticular disease to avoid eating nuts, popcorn, seeds, and even foods like tomatoes that have tiny seeds inside. They were worried these little hard nuggets might cause intestinal damage or bleeding.

But when researchers tested this idea, they found the opposite may be true. A study in the prestigious *Journal of the American Medical Association* found that men who ate more nuts, popcorn, and corn were less likely to develop intestinal complications or bleeding.

It's possible the nutrients and fiber in these foods helped keep their intestines healthy. Ask your doctor if it's safe for you to enjoy popcorn and nuts again.

HEALTH ALERT!

Common pain relievers may raise your risk of diverticular disease. Researchers followed a group of 47,000 men for 22 years, keeping track of what drugs they took and who developed diverticulitis or intestinal bleeding. Those who took aspirin or other nonsteroidal anti-inflammatory drugs (NSAIDs) regularly — between two and six times per week — had the highest risk of diverticulitis.

Esophageal cancer

Safeguard your esophagus with strawberries

Americans only eat around 8 pounds of strawberries a year, but legend has it that Madame Tallien of Napoleon's court used 22 pounds of strawberries in just one bath. This doesn't mean you should start bathing in strawberries. But experts suggest eating more strawberries might help reduce your risk of cancer of the esophagus.

Esophageal cancer develops in the tube that carries food, liquid, and saliva from your mouth to your stomach. It is one of the leading causes of cancer deaths around the world. More than 22,000 new cases appear in the United States every year, and even more occur in China.

That is why Ohio State University researchers recruited 75 people in China who had already developed precancerous lesions on the esophagus. The researchers graded each precancerous area from low grade with less danger of cancer to higher grades with a greater cancer risk.

The researchers also divided the study participants into two groups. Group 1 took an ounce of freeze-dried strawberries with a little water once a day for six months, while Group 2 took the same amount twice a day. The extra dose of strawberries made a difference. At the end of the study, the precancerous lesions of most Group 2 members had improved and were less likely to become cancerous.

Be aware that this study was funded by the California Strawberry Commission, and a dose of freeze-dried strawberries is 10 times more concentrated than the same amount of fresh strawberries. But the study's lead researcher says you can still benefit from eating fresh strawberries.

Earlier animal research with freeze-dried black raspberries, strawberries, and blackberries also suggests berries may help prevent esophageal cancer.

The scientists say more research is needed to find out whether berries can help prevent esophageal cancer. But meanwhile, it's still a good idea to eat a serving of berries every day. Eat fresh berries as a snack, add them to smoothies or salads, or use them to top your yogurt and hot or cold cereal.

HEALTH ALERT!

Research from China and the Middle East found that drinking warm green or black tea is safe, but your odds of esophageal cancer go up if your tea is 140 degrees or higher when you sip it.

People who drank tea below this temperature, or waited at least four minutes for the tea to cool, had significantly less risk of this deadly cancer. Hot liquids and foods can injure the cells lining your esophagus, causing inflammation that can lead to cancer.

What's more, a 10-year study of older adults found that those who ate the most red meat had a higher risk of cancer of the esophagus. If you eat red meat every day, cut back to twice a week to protect yourself. Substitute poultry or fish on other days.

Fatigue

Energize your diet with smart food combos

You feel tired and irritable. Sometimes it seems you just can't catch your breath, and there's no good explanation for your headaches and weakness. The problem may be anemia, a deficiency of iron in your blood. Some 10 percent of people 65 years and older suffer from anemia, and the rate jumps up to 60 percent for those in nursing homes. That puts them at higher risk for falls.

Your body needs iron to carry oxygen to muscles and other cells, so if you don't have enough you may feel tired and weak. Most people get enough iron from eating meat, eggs, enriched cereals, and even vegetables like beans and greens.

Pump up the volume. If you're trying to cut down on meat, you'll need to use a few tricks to make sure your body is getting enough iron. That's because this nutrient comes in two forms — heme, which you get from meat, and nonheme, which comes from plant sources.

It's easy for your body to absorb heme iron. But that's not the case with nonheme iron. Fortunately, you can boost the amount your body gets by eating foods rich in vitamin C or protein with your meals, since both of these nutrients improve the absorption of nonheme iron.

> People who get their heme iron from red meat are more likely to develop metabolic syndrome, marked by problems with weight, blood pressure, cholesterol, triglycerides, and blood sugar.

So plan food pairings like pinto beans stewed with tomatoes and onions, or rice with sauteed broccoli. Mixing sliced strawberries into a bowl of fortified oatmeal also does the trick.

Steer clear of supplements. If you have trouble with low iron, you may want to avoid polyphenol supplements like grape seed extract or EGCG from green tea. These healthy polyphenols can block iron absorption in your intestines — just what you don't want.

HEALTH ALERT!

Your fingernails can tell you a lot about your health. Pale, white nail beds can be a sign of iron deficiency anemia. It's a condition called koilonychia, and you may also notice your nails have a concave shape, or spoon shape. The edges of your nails may be raised and thin.

But nail changes like these can also occur if you use petroleum-based solvents on the job or if your nail has been injured. There's also an inherited condition that causes similar misshaped nails. Ask your doctor about doing a blood test to see what your nails are really saying.

Morning pick-me-up that never fails

Even if you're a morning person, you can feel sluggish and slow when the alarm clock sounds. Put a spring in your step by starting your day with a glass of water. More powerful than a strong cup of coffee, a glass of water before breakfast can put an end to morning dehydration and get you ready for the day. Here's why.

Overnight fasting dries you out. You've been sleeping all night, and you need to replenish that 60 percent of your body that's made of water. When you get dehydrated, your metabolic rate goes down. That can make you feel lethargic and low in energy.

Water boosts your nervous system. This drink does more than just cure your thirst. It also boosts the activity of your sympathetic nervous system — the fight-or-flight reaction that keeps you alert and ready for action.

Fluids keep blood pressure even. You may feel faint — or even find yourself passing out — when your body needs water. Researchers believe the connection between water and dizziness is related to not having enough blood volume in your veins to keep it flowing smoothly. Because blood is about 80 percent water, it's at the mercy of your drinking habits. That's one reason why you should have a drink when you donate blood.

> Water can also regulate weight. One expert calculated you might shed up to 5 pounds a year just by drinking three glasses of water a day.

A program in England encouraging seniors to drink more water through the day was a great success. After just a week or two of

Did you know?

You can't rely on feeling thirsty to know when you should drink more water. The sense of thirst may drop as you get older, and some drugs can make you dehydrated before you know it.

But you also may not need to chug down eight glasses of water a day to be sure you get enough fluids. Remember that you get about 20 percent of the water you need from foods, such as citrus fruits and soup. Of the remaining 80 percent, some can come from beverages other than plain water.

Aim to meet your fluid needs by enjoying low-fat milk, unsweetened tea, and some real fruit juice, along with water.

following new habits, seniors said they had more energy, were steadier on their feet, had fewer bladder problems, and generally felt better. That's a lot gained from a small effort.

Sniff the right scents to stay alert

Nothing makes you feel tired and cranky like a long, tedious drive on the highway. A little aromatherapy may help ease the discomfort and help you stay awake.

A research team from West Virginia tested how drivers reacted to the scents of cinnamon, peppermint, or nothing at all. They found that drivers who enjoyed either cinnamon or peppermint scents felt more alert and less fatigued and frustrated while on the road. Meanwhile, those who had no special scent added to their environment felt no different.

The researchers say these scents may help to stimulate the central nervous system, so they can boost your performance, motivation, and alertness while lessening exhaustion while you drive. Equipping your car with a bit of cinnamon potpourri or a peppermint sachet is certainly a simpler way to stay awake than loading up on coffee or energy drinks.

> Some people swear by a stick of cinnamon chewing gum or a peppermint breath mint to keep them awake and refreshed during a boring task.

Aromatherapy works by delivering specific scents through essential oils that may be diluted and applied to your skin or sprayed in the air. But never place undiluted essential oils directly on your skin. Dilute them first in a carrier oil.

Boost your energy with beets

Belly up to the salad bar, and choose a cheery red vegetable to raise your energy level and improve your muscle function. Beets are one selection you may be ignoring, but their natural supply of nitrates helps your muscles work harder.

Researchers knew eating foods naturally high in nitrates, like beets and spinach, could bring down your blood pressure. That's because your body converts nitrates from food into nitric oxide, which dilates blood vessels to let your blood flow smoothly.

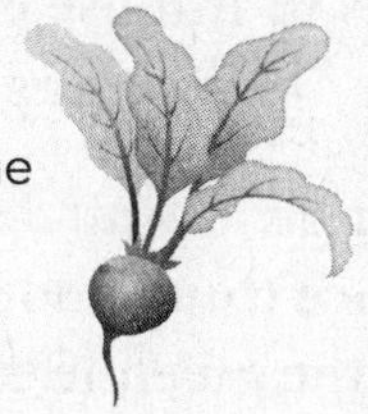

A bumper crop of beets is a good thing, but you can't eat them all at once. Spread the bounty of beets over weeks and months by eating some now and preparing some for later. Here's how to use and preserve these ruby treats.

- Use fresh beets on salad. Grate raw beets and sprinkle them on a tossed salad. Eating beets fresh and uncooked may give you more antioxidants.
- Roast and preserve beets. Mix sliced beets and tomatoes and roast them in the oven, then put them in a jar with a little olive oil. The mixture will keep well in the refrigerator.
- Dry beets for safe storage. Roast beets until nearly done, then slice them into small, uniformly sized pieces. Then bake the beet slices in a single layer on a baking sheet. Turn as needed. When they're crispy, they're done.

But nitric oxide in your blood has other benefits, so researchers tested how it might boost exercise performance. They compared beetroot juice with blackcurrant juice, a fruit drink that's low in nitrates. Eight adults drank about 17 ounces of juice daily, then took part in high-intensity cycling exercise.

After 15 days of drinking beetroot juice, the people in the study had higher levels of nitric oxide in their blood, making them more efficient at using oxygen. That let them work harder during exercise tests without needing more oxygen to fuel their muscles. If you've ever had to stop and catch your breath while chasing your dog, you know how oxygen use relates to intense exercise. But when folks drank beetroot juice, it was "hello energy, goodbye fatigue."

Other great sources of nitrates include spinach and celery. But the nice thing about beets is they're also high in potassium — both the green leafy part and the red roots. Some experts say a lack of potassium may also leave you feeling weak and lacking in energy. And beets have other health benefits as well. To learn more, see "Beet juice beats dementia" in the *Alzheimer's and memory loss* chapter.

Fibromyalgia

No-fuss way to cut the pain

Experts say some 4 million U.S. adults are living with fibromyalgia. This chronic condition makes you feel pain all over — especially in specific tender spots — so weak and tired you can't function normally, and unable to sleep. You may also suffer from headaches, depression, and trouble thinking.

Certain drugs battle fibromyalgia symptoms, but research shows you can also get some relief from what you drink. Tart cherry juice, with its anti-inflammatory and antioxidant powers, may help your muscles and your whole body stay strong and pain-free.

Cut fibromyalgia pain. In one study, women with fibromyalgia who drank 10.5 ounces of tart cherry juice twice daily for 10 days had less pain. They also kept up their muscle strength even after researchers had them do challenging arm exercises. The results shouldn't be surprising, since tart cherry juice was already successful in stopping oxidative damage in seniors who did similar exercise tests.

Improve sleep. Tart cherry juice also has lots of melatonin, a natural hormone that regulates your sleep-wake cycle. That's important, since fibromyalgia can crush your ability to get a good night's rest. Researchers found that people who enjoyed a glass of cherry juice twice a day slept longer at night and napped less during the day.

Help muscles recover. Anthocyanins in tart cherry juice are also known to cut post-exercise pain. These antioxidant compounds give the juice color and help lower inflammation. Researchers found that runners taking part in a long-distance race had less soreness and muscle pain after the race if they drank tart cherry juice for several days before the event.

You could get similar benefits from eating whole Montmorency cherries, but you would need to eat 90 to 100 whole cherries to get the same benefit as you get from 1 ounce of tart cherry juice concentrate. So drink up and enjoy.

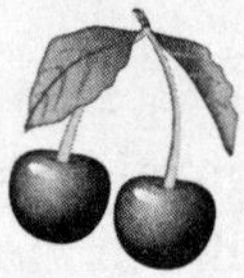

Drinking tart cherry juice is not as expensive a solution for your fibromyalgia symptoms as you may think. You have two basic options.

- Buy ready-to-drink tart cherry juice. A brand like Indian Summer Montmorency tart cherry juice comes in 46-ounce bottles. It costs around 70 cents for an 8-ounce serving.
- Buy concentrated cherry juice, then mix 2 tablespoons into an 8-ounce glass of water. Tart Is Smart tart cherry juice concentrate sells for around 90 cents per 8-ounce serving.

Relieve pain with pumpkin seeds

Instead of popping a pain pill, try popping a handful of pumpkin seeds. These tasty treats are jam-packed with magnesium — just the mineral that may battle fibromyalgia pain.

An ounce of roasted pumpkin seeds provides 156 milligrams (mg) of magnesium. That's a lot, considering senior women should get 320 mg a day, while older men require 420 mg. Researchers found that giving people with fibromyalgia supplements of magnesium along with malic acid, a natural substance found in some fruits, helped reduce their pain and tenderness. The supplements contained just 50 mg of magnesium, so you're getting three times that amount in a handful of pumpkin seeds.

Other research has found that middle-aged women with fibromyalgia have significantly lower levels of minerals, including magnesium, than healthy women — and that taking magnesium supplements may help with pain and other symptoms.

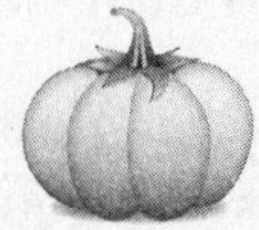

Of course you can roast pumpkin seeds, but you can also boil, microwave, or dehydrate these autumn favorites. Drying them gives a result very different from roasting, and they'll be ready to use in trail mix or granola.

First wash the seeds to remove pumpkin flesh. To dry the seeds in a food dehydrator, set the temperature to 115 to 120 degrees Fahrenheit for one to two hours. You can also put them on a baking sheet in a warm oven for three or four hours. Stir seeds often so they don't burn.

Meatless diet can make life brighter

Focusing on plant-based foods in your diet can stave off lots of chronic health problems, and fibromyalgia is no exception. Researchers tested a strict vegetarian diet on a group of 30 people with fibromyalgia for seven months. Nearly two-thirds enjoyed a better quality of life, less shoulder and neck pain and stiffness, and better sleep while following the meatless diet.

Participants in the study didn't change anything in their lives except what they were eating. The researchers told them to keep using any pain or sleep medicines they were already taking. However, changes to their diets were drastic, including cutting out all meat and dairy products along with caffeine and alcohol. In fact, not everyone was willing to stay on the plan. But it's just these big changes that led to improvement.

Because people in the study were eating lots of fresh fruits and vegetables, the high levels of antioxidants, phytochemicals, and detoxification enzymes they were getting might be expected to change their body processes. But the researchers aren't really sure exactly what elements in the diet helped. They suggest that simply being able to take action and help themselves may account for some of the improvements. In addition, sleeping better might have helped their overall outlook on life.

The vegetarian diet included about 85 percent raw foods, with 15 percent cooked. The basic plan looks like this.

- Eat lots of fresh fruits and green salads, along with nuts, seeds, legumes, and whole grains.
- Include flaxseed oil and extra virgin olive oil in place of hydrogenated oils.
- Avoid caffeine, alcohol, refined sugar and flour, dairy, eggs, and all meats.
- Eat steamed or stir-fried vegetables, baked potatoes and sweet potatoes, and freshly prepared soups.
- Drink herb teas, organic juices, and a small amount of almond milk and rice milk.
- Sweeten foods naturally with honey, unsulphured molasses, pure maple syrup, stevia, date sugar, or agave nectar.

For more tips on how a vegetarian diet can improve your health, see "Nature's all-natural cataract preventers" in the *Vision loss* chapter and "Cut meat to curb belly pain" in the *Diverticulitis* chapter.

Food poisoning

Steer clear of these foods

Every year, about 1 in 6 Americans suffers from food poisoning. Foodborne bacteria, like *Salmonella* and *E. coli*, kill some 3,000 people annually, so it's no minor problem. In fact, research shows that a serious bout of food poisoning may have long-term effects, including higher risks for kidney failure, arthritis, diabetes, nerve damage, and high blood pressure.

Everyone knows eating raw oysters can be risky, but dangerous pathogens may also lurk in common "healthy" foods.

Undercooked beef and poultry. Deadly bacteria including *E. coli, Staphylococcus*, and others may lurk in raw hamburger or chicken. Use a meat thermometer to cook chicken to at least 165 degrees Fahrenheit inside, and don't indulge in rare cheeseburgers.

Unpasteurized dairy, eggs, and juice. Milk, cheese, eggs, and even fruit juices are pasteurized to kill harmful bacteria. Fans of "raw" milk and other untreated foods forego this risk-reducing process to consume potentially dangerous products, thinking it's healthier for them. But raw milk causes three times the hospitalizations of any other type of foodborne illness.

Unwashed greens, sprouts, and fruit. Norovirus lurking in fresh greens, salad mixes, and fruit has caused some of the largest outbreaks of produce-related illnesses. Other widespread outbreaks have been caused by deadly *Salmonella* in tomatoes, sprouts, and melons. Cross-contamination from animal waste or improper food handling are usually to blame. Scrub melons with mild dishwashing liquid before you cut them open, and rinse off lettuce leaves under running water before you eat them.

HEALTH ALERT!

Don't eat raw cookie dough — an outbreak of *E. coli* infection was caused by raw cookie dough bought from the supermarket. Even though the dough contained instructions to bake it before eating, customers couldn't resist.

Both homemade and store-bought raw dough may contain raw eggs, a possible carrier of dangerous bacteria. It turned out the tainted product in this case had flour contaminated with *E. coli.*

Spice up your quest for food safety

Add a little more cilantro to your homemade salsa. Better yet, add a lot. This fiesta favorite is known to kill many types of foodborne bacteria, including *E. coli, Salmonella*, and *Staphylococcus*. It also adds great flavor to your southwestern dishes.

Researchers have tested both coriander oil, from the same plant, and natural chemicals isolated from the herb to see what effects they have on bacteria. A dozen strains of bacteria, including common types known to cause food poisoning, were slowed or killed by a weak solution of cilantro extracts. The researchers found that bacteria suffered damage to their cell membranes, leading to their death.

You can spice up your cooking using the dried seeds and fresh leaves of the cilantro plant. Both contain high levels of dodecenal, a natural compound found to be twice as effective at killing *Salmonella* as the antibiotic gentamicin. Cilantro also contains other helpful phytonutrients, including quercetin and caffeic acid, which may protect cells from oxidative damage.

Fresh cilantro is available in the grocery store all year, and it's one of the main ingredients in fresh salsa, along with tomatoes, onions, and chilies. You can also store whole dried coriander seeds for up to a year.

Did you know?

Rumor has it that Twinkies can last forever due to their high levels of preservatives. But they only stay fresh for 20 days. However, there is one delicious treat with an expiration date you don't have to worry about.

All natural honey may be good nearly forever. Its antibiotic properties keep it from spoiling. Honey may crystallize over time, but it's still good to eat. Simply place the jar in warm water, and stir the honey to dissolve the crystals. Then go ahead and enjoy it in your tea, on toast, or as a natural sweetener.

Sprinkle on a dash of defense

Humble spices like cinnamon and cloves do more than add flavor. They can also stop food poisoning by killing bacteria and stopping the growth of fungus in foods.

Keep ground beef safe. *Escherichia coli (E. coli)* is a dangerous bacterium that can cause severe diarrhea and flu-like symptoms. It likes to hide in partially cooked meats and unpasteurized foods, like fresh apple cider. Previous research showed when cinnamon was added to apple juice infected with *E. coli*, the cinnamon killed more than 99 percent of the bacteria after three days.

Other studies show cinnamon and other spices are effective in killing *E. coli* in ground beef. Researchers at Kansas State University found cinnamon — along with cloves, garlic, oregano, and sage — keeps *E. coli* from growing in raw beef and salami. Researchers in Japan had similar results with spices tested in the lab. They believe that eugenol, an oil that can be extracted from cinnamon and other spices, is what battles the deadly bacteria.

Don't be fooled by names. You may see cilantro referred to as coriander, Chinese parsley, or dhania. It's all the same herb.

Help bread last longer. Over in Spain, researchers found that infusing waxed paper with cinnamon essential oil, then wrapping sliced bread in this paper, could stop the growth of mold. The bread had been infected with mold spores, so it should have been fuzzy and inedible pretty quickly. But even after three days, it appeared the cinnamon oil blocked mold growth and kept the bread fresh.

Even the experts don't know how much cinnamon it takes to keep food safe, so don't give up following safe food-handling practices just yet. The U.S. Centers for Disease Control and Prevention recommends these steps:

- Wash your hands often.
- Keep raw food separate from ready-to-eat food.
- Cook foods to the proper temperatures.
- Refrigerate leftovers promptly.
- Report foodborne illness to your local health department.

Spicy cinnamon steak rub

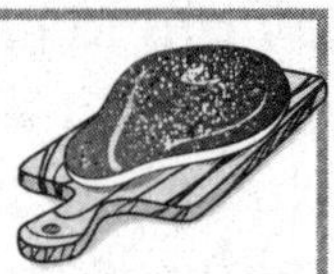

Put cinnamon to work on your steak by including it in a dry rub. Blend together the following spices, then rub the mixture evenly on all sides of 2 pounds of New York strip steaks. Cover and refrigerate for 20 minutes, then grill or broil the steaks until done to your liking.

1 1/2 teaspoons ground cinnamon

1 teaspoon paprika

1 teaspoon oregano

1/2 teaspoon garlic powder

1/2 teaspoon salt

1/4 teaspoon ground red pepper

2 teaspoons brown sugar

GERD

Foods that help and foods that hurt

Prevent heartburn without making a trip to the drugstore. Discover common heartburn "trigger foods" — and the foods that will fight against reflux disease and cancer. Which ones are on your plate?

Everyone may experience heartburn or indigestion from time to time. But if you have gastroesophageal reflux disease (GERD), you experience it frequently.

Acid reflux happens when stomach acid flows back into your esophagus, the tube that carries food, liquid, and saliva from your mouth to your stomach. The lower esophageal sphincter, the muscle that serves as a valve between your esophagus and stomach, seems to be the culprit. If it weakens or relaxes, stomach acid flows into your esophagus.

This acid backwash irritates your esophagus and causes symptoms. The main symptom is heartburn — the burning sensation behind your breastbone — but you may also have a cough or trouble swallowing. GERD can seriously damage the lining of your esophagus. Long-term irritation may contribute to the changes in cells that cause esophageal cancer.

Before resorting to medication to treat GERD, try some lifestyle changes. Losing weight and quitting smoking can help. So can the following dietary tips.

Set aside the saltshaker. Adding table salt to your food can boost your risk of GERD by a whopping 70 percent, according to a Norwegian study. People who always added extra salt to their meals increased their risk just as much as those who smoked daily for at least 20 years.

Feast on fiber. The same study found a protective effect for fiber. People who regularly ate high-fiber breads essentially sliced their risk of GERD in half compared to those who preferred low-fiber white bread. Fiber has previously been found to reduce the risk of esophageal and stomach cancers. Researchers speculate that fiber may work by scavenging nitrites in the stomach, lowering the amount of nitric oxide produced. Nitric oxide may relax the lower esophageal sphincter, leading to acid reflux.

Tiptoe around triggers. Besides salt, you may want to cut back on foods that may worsen your heartburn symptoms. These traditional triggers include acidic foods like tomatoes and citrus fruits, fatty or fried foods, spicy foods, caffeine, alcohol, carbonated beverages, garlic, onions, mint, and chocolate. Although doctors traditionally recommend avoiding these foods, research does not always support this tactic. Still, it's worth experimenting by eliminating certain foods to see if your symptoms clear up.

Good news for coffee lovers

You enjoy drinking coffee, but not the heartburn that follows. Switching to a dark-roasted coffee could help. Researchers discovered that dark-roasted coffee contains a compound that helps reduce stomach acid.

Called N-methylpyridinium (NMP), this compound is generated only with roasting. So dark-roasted coffee contains more of it — up to twice as much as light-roasted varieties. Unlike NMP, caffeine helps stimulate the secretion of stomach acid. So a decaffeinated, dark-roasted coffee might be your best bet.

Tap into turmeric's healing powers

Turmeric adds a glorious shade of gold to your tasty curries and stews. But this aromatic spice's powers don't stop there. Long valued as a traditional medicine, natural compounds in turmeric have been found to slow unwanted hair growth, cleanse wounds, and help neutralize cobra venom.

One of those compounds — a polyphenol called curcumin — acts as a strong antioxidant and anti-inflammatory. Those powers may prove essential in the treatment of gastroesophageal reflux disease (GERD).

One study designed to mimic the effects of stomach acid backwash on people with GERD found that curcumin blocked cytokine activity in esophageal cells. How does that help? Cytokines are powerful proteins known to cause inflammation.

Scientists also looked at how curcumin might help people with Barrett's esophagus — a condition in which GERD causes abnormal cellular changes to the lining of the lower esophagus. Those changes are thought to increase the risk of developing cancer.

The researchers found that a daily dose of 500 milligrams of curcumin over seven days doubled the frequency of apoptosis — that is, the rate at which dysfunctional cells die on schedule — in people with Barrett's esophagus. Why is that good? One of the hallmarks of cancer is the ability of abnormal cells to evade apoptosis, divide without control, and invade surrounding tissue or spread to other parts of the body.

Put heartburn to rest with melatonin

Suffering from heartburn? Melatonin may provide relief. You probably think of melatonin as the sleep hormone, but it also plays an important role in digestive health. In fact, evidence suggests that melatonin may be an effective treatment for gastroesophageal reflux disease (GERD) — with fewer side effects than commonly prescribed drugs.

In one study, a Brazilian researcher compared a combination of melatonin and other nutrients to omeprazole, a proton pump inhibitor often used to treat GERD symptoms. The supplement included 6 milligrams (mg) of melatonin, plus tryptophan, vitamin B6, vitamin B12, methionine, folic acid, and betaine.

After 40 days, all 176 people in the melatonin group reported relief of symptoms, compared to just two-thirds of those in the omeprazole group. After the study, the 60 people in the omeprazole group who did not respond to the drug switched to the melatonin blend for 40 days — and all of them found relief.

Melatonin may work by preventing the secretion of stomach acid and by stopping the lower esophageal sphincter, the valve between the stomach and esophagus, from relaxing at the wrong time.

The recommended amount to soothe heartburn is 6 mg of melatonin taken around bedtime. Experts suggest sticking with your normal GERD medications for the first 40 days of melatonin treatment. After that, keep a dose of your regular medication on hand, and take it whenever symptoms reappear. If you are taking a prescription drug to relieve your symptoms, check with your doctor before trying melatonin.

As a bonus, melatonin should help you sleep. That's important because GERD is a common cause of sleep problems, and certain sleeping pills may worsen symptoms. Other ways to improve your sleep if you have GERD include elevating the head of your bed and sleeping on your left side.

Reduce heartburn with this trick

Don't grab an antacid for occasional heartburn. Reach for a tasty alternative instead. A stick of chewing gum will give you fast relief. It gets your saliva flowing, which helps neutralize backed-up stomach acid and wash it away naturally.

Try it yourself. Next time you have heartburn, chew sugar-free gum for half an hour. Peppermint can trigger this condition, so avoid that flavor.

Healthy mouth & teeth

Reel in healthy gums to prevent tooth loss

Keep your pearly whites longer by adding fish to your meals. Researchers found that people who eat more fish — specifically, those who get more polyunsaturated fats like those in fish — are about 20 percent less likely to develop periodontitis, or gum disease. This chronic inflammation of your gums can lead to tooth loss. That's why it's important to stop it before it's too late.

More than 9,000 people who were part of the National Health and Nutrition Examination Survey (NHANES) answered questions about what they ate. They also had dental exams to check for gum disease. People who reported eating more omega-3 fatty acids were less likely to show signs of gum disease.

Both docosahexaenoic acid (DHA) and eicosapentaenoic acid (EPA), omega-3s found in fatty fish, were linked with protection from gum disease. Eating more vegetable fats, like alpha-linolenic acid (ALA), did not seem to make a difference. The experts suspect the omega-3 fatty acids in fish decrease inflammation by targeting the bacteria responsible for gum disease.

People who ate the greatest amount of healthy fats didn't have any more protection than those who ate a moderate amount, so you don't need to go overboard with fish dinners to get gum protection. Simply follow the same goals for fish eating that the American Heart Association recommends to help your heart — two servings of fish, particularly fatty fish like salmon or herring, a week.

Try this easy brushing trick

You need a bit of extra elbow grease to scrub away food bits that are stuck to your dishes. So wouldn't the same reasoning apply to getting your teeth squeaky clean?

No — brushing harder won't do your mouth any favors. In fact, it may have the opposite effect. Experts warn that vigorous brushing may increase your risk of bleeding and receding gums. And it may even cause the enamel on your teeth to wear away, leading to cavities and other painful problems.

Instead, brush gently with a soft-bristled toothbrush to cut down on plaque. Angle your brush so that it is at a 45-degree angle to your gumline. Use short, gentle strokes.

Yogurt — a tasty treat that's good for your mouth

The same natural yogurt that keeps your digestion running smoothly also helps your mouth in three big ways.

Fights bad breath. Eating plain yogurt can clean your mouth of hydrogen sulfide, a bad-smelling compound that contributes to halitosis, or bad breath. Researchers found this trick worked for 80 percent of people who chowed down on 3.5 ounces of yogurt twice daily. Pick sugarless yogurt with live active cultures, which fights the bacteria that lead to bad breath.

Keeps teeth and gums healthy. A survey of people middle-aged and older found those who ate more lactic acid foods tended to have less gum disease. Researchers looked at signs of gum disease, including pocket depth around teeth and loss of attachment between gums and teeth. These are signs that gum disease is getting worse, and your teeth may be at risk. Folks with more advanced gum disease reported eating less lactic acid food on a regular basis.

4 ways to get more yogurt in your day

Use low-fat yogurt in your recipes in place of high-fat ingredients, and you can enjoy more calcium and protein in every meal. Greek yogurt is strained and concentrated, so it contains higher levels of probiotics and more protein than many regular yogurts. Try these kitchen substitutions.

- Make a marinade of yogurt and spices, and use it for steaks or chicken.
- Replace sour cream with yogurt when you create salad dressings or dips.
- Whip up creamy mashed potatoes with a scoop of yogurt folded in.
- Blend together fruit-flavored yogurt, strawberries, and blueberries for a berry smoothie.

If you eat yogurt and drink kefir or buttermilk, you're getting lactic acid foods. Eating them helps fight the bacteria that lead to plaque buildup in your mouth. Other research has found that strains of helpful bacteria called probiotics can cut the plaque in your mouth and improve signs of gum disease.

Dairy foods like yogurt, milk, and cheese also provide calcium to build strong bones and teeth.

Blocks canker sores. Those annoying and painful mouth sores may also respond to the probiotic effects of real yogurt. Experts say applying powdered cultures of *Lactobacillus acidophilus* or *Lactobacillus bulgaricus* directly to your mouth sores twice a day may help them heal faster. These probiotics are available in pills and capsules at drugstores or online. You can also get some forms of *Lactobacillus* from eating yogurt with live active cultures.

Say 'cheese' for healthier teeth

Eating a morsel of cheese after dinner or as a snack between meals can help cut tooth decay. Along with providing minerals like calcium and phosphorus that strengthen tooth enamel, cheese encourages saliva production and neutralizes acids in your mouth. So join in the European tradition of ending a meal with cheese, and impress your dentist.

Another benefit — if you add high-fat, hard cheese to your diet, your LDL cholesterol — the bad kind — may not go up like it would if you piled on the butter. Researchers think this difference is due to the high content of calcium in cheese.

> Want to spice up your food and protect your pearly whites? Then consider adding a dab of horseradish to your meals. Some say this spicy paste has enzymes that can fight off the bacteria that cause tooth decay. Horseradish gives a fiery kick to eggs, hummus, and even tomato soup. Or add a spoonful to your favorite dip or salad dressing for extra flavor.

All-natural breath fresheners

Here's a folk remedy you can really chew on. Pick one of these all-natural herbal breath "mints" from your kitchen, and chew them with or after meals. People around the world swear by them for fresh breath.

- parsley
- oregano
- dill
- mint
- fennel seeds
- anise seeds
- cinnamon
- cardamom
- basil
- thyme

Sip green tea for fresh breath

Fill your cup with green tea and you'll be surprised how drinking it freshens your breath.

Experts already knew the polyphenols in green tea kill mouth bacteria in the lab, but they wanted to see how green tea might work in people. So they devised a study to test how green tea cuts the bad-smelling volatile sulfur compounds that cause bad breath. Volatile sulfur compounds include hydrogen sulfide, which smells like rotten eggs, and methyl mercaptan, which has a rotten cabbage odor. Byproducts from your body's breakdown of protein and fat can cause these odors. That's why people who eat meat are more likely to have bad breath than vegetarians.

Researchers compared green tea with popular remedies people rely on to curb bad breath. Men in the study first had their breath analyzed for bad smells, then either brushed their teeth with Crest toothpaste, chewed gum, sucked on mints, or ate parsley supplements. Another group swished around green tea powder and then swallowed. The powder was chosen because it provides a standardized amount of green tea.

At one, two, and three hours after the bad breath remedies, researchers checked for sulfur compounds in the men's breath. Turns out green tea worked better than the other remedies at fighting bad breath. But even green tea only worked for a while. After three hours, the effects had worn off.

You can take your green tea the old-fashioned way — brewed in a cup. But drink it unsweetened, and swish it around your mouth before you swallow.

After you've finished drinking a cup of green tea, use the leftover tea bag to soothe sore and painful gums. After steeping the bag, let it cool, and hold it on the affected area.

Did you know?

Chewing gum is a tried-and-true way to sweeten bad breath. That's because it leads to more saliva production, which helps wash away bacteria and food particles.

Choose a cinnamon gum like Big Red for even more breath protection. Cinnamic aldehyde, the natural compound that gives cinnamon its unique flavor and smell, blocks the growth of mouth bacteria that cause bad breath.

Gluten sensitivity linked to mouth sores

Get tested for gluten intolerance if you get canker sores over and over again, especially if the usual treatments don't work. Some people who are sensitive to gluten, a protein found in wheat and other grains, can cure their sores by avoiding it.

You may know of gluten sensitivity as the root of celiac disease, an autoimmune condition that causes damage to your intestinal lining. But researchers found you can have gluten sensitivity and show only one sign — mouth sores. They tested the blood of 247 people with recurrent canker sores to check for antibodies to gluten. A small number had antibodies. Those folks were told to follow a gluten-free diet, and their mouth sores cleared up in a matter of months.

Even without symptoms, however, a gluten intolerance could be doing damage to your intestines. If you have mouth sores that appear more than three times a year, ask your doctor about being tested for gluten sensitivity.

Here's how to avoid gluten.

- Don't eat foods that contain wheat, rye, barley, malt, or oats. Although oats are actually gluten-free, they can be contaminated if they are processed in the same plant with other grains. That means most foods made from grains — breads, pasta, crackers, cookies — are off limits.

- Check food labels for the words "gluten free." If you don't see them, read the list of ingredients.
- Look for gluten-free substitutes for your favorite foods, like pasta made from brown rice, corn, or quinoa.
- Beware of gluten from unexpected sources, like communion wafers, medicine, lipstick, canned foods, luncheon meats, candy, and ice cream.

Get help for canker sores

When pain from a canker sore keeps you from eating or talking, you want it gone fast. Experts have developed patches you can put on canker sores and leave in place to stop the pain and speed healing.

The Canker Cover patch covers your sore so nothing acidic or salty can irritate it. Natural ingredients, including menthol, xylitol, and citrus oil, block pain and help it heal. Another brand, CankerMelts, works in a similar way, but its natural ingredients include licorice.

Research shows the patches can give relief from canker sores. Look for these natural patches at your local supermarket or drugstore.

Take a coffee break to dodge mouth cancer

Your morning cuppa Joe may help protect you from cancers of the mouth and throat. Researchers found that the heaviest coffee drinkers — people who usually have a third and fourth cup of caffeinated coffee daily — were 39 percent less likely to suffer from one of these cancers.

The researchers looked at several studies of people in the United States, Europe, and Central America, checking to see what they ate and drank and who tended to develop cancers of the mouth and throat. They examined the habits of about 14,000 people, some with cancer and some cancer-free. People who drank at least 4 cups of coffee a day had the lowest risk of mouth and throat cancers, but the same was not true for people who drank decaffeinated coffee or any kind of tea.

It's still unclear how caffeinated coffee may help prevent cancer, but experts say it's probably due to its more than 1,000 natural chemicals. These include phenols like caffeic and ferulic acids, along with chemicals in the diterpene family that may trigger enzymes involved in blocking cancer.

Other research has hinted that coffee drinking may also protect from cancers of the colon, liver, prostate, and skin.

Tea extract targets precancerous sores

People who have already suffered from oral leukoplakia — precancerous mouth sores — may benefit from green tea extract. Researchers found that more than half of people at risk who took green tea extract three times a day for three months showed increased protection. As with other benefits of green tea, antioxidant polyphenols get the credit for protection. In this case, they seem to stop the development of tumors.

Side effects were mild. Those taking the highest dose, which was equal to drinking 24 cups of green tea a day, had some nervousness and trouble sleeping.

Hearing loss

Protect your hearing with beans

It sounds too good to be true, but a B vitamin may actually reduce hearing loss in old age. This B vitamin is called folate, vitamin B9, and sometimes folic acid. And exciting research from around the world confirms why you need it to protect your hearing.

- People age 50 or older who had the lowest blood levels of folate were 39 percent more likely to have hearing loss, Australian researchers discovered. The researchers also checked blood levels of the amino acid homocysteine, because high homocysteine levels have been linked with low folate. They found that people with the highest levels of homocysteine had a 64 percent higher risk of developing hearing loss than people with normal homocysteine levels.
- Boston researchers evaluated the hearing and intake of vitamins C, E, beta carotene, B12, and folate for more than 26,000 men. Among men age 60 or older, those who took in the most folate from food or supplements had a 20 percent lower risk of hearing loss than men who took in the least folate.
- Healthy people over age 60 who have age-related hearing loss are more likely to have low blood levels of folate than people with normal hearing, a Nigerian study reported.

Low levels of folate and high levels of homocysteine can be bad news for your cochlea, a spiral shaped chamber in your inner ear that is vital to your hearing. Your cochlea needs a good blood supply from a large number of blood vessels in order to do its job. Unfortunately, homocysteine can damage those blood vessels. Animal research suggests high homocysteine can also damage the cochlea in other ways.

Both blood vessel disease and problems with the cochlea have been linked with hearing loss. That is why experts think excessive homocysteine may be bad for both your cochlea and your hearing. Because a shortage of folate leads to too much homocysteine, making sure you get enough folate may be a smart way to help protect your hearing.

Fortunately, adding more folate to your diet is not hard. Enjoy these five delicious, inexpensive, easy-to-find foods that are just brimming with it.

Food	Percent of DRI in a cup
lentils	90%
pinto beans	74%
chickpeas or garbanzo beans	71%
black beans	64%
navy beans	64%

Relieve the ringing in your ears

Ringing in the ears happens to most people every once in awhile. But for some 20 million Americans with chronic tinnitus, that ringing happens frequently and interferes with daily living.

If you notice a constant or recurring ringing in your ears that has lasted six months or more, see your doctor. Other persistent noises like buzzing, hissing, roaring, humming, shrieking, or chirping may also be signs of tinnitus.

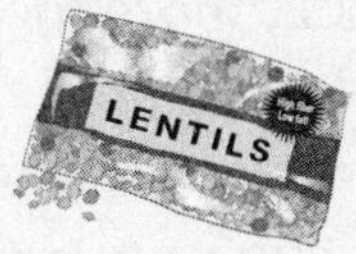

Good news if you've never tried brown lentils before. These legumes don't require soaking before you use them. Just sort out any debris or small stones and rinse. To cook lentils, bring 3 cups of water, chicken broth, or vegetable broth to a boil in a large pot. Stir in 1 cup of lentils, and briefly bring to a boil again. Let simmer for 20 minutes. When they are tender, they are done.

To prevent digestive problems, always bring the cooking liquid to a boil before adding the lentils.

For an easy, delicious dish, spread a layer of cooked lentils over a layer of cooked brown rice. Top with caramelized onions and plain, unsweetened yogurt.

Sometimes tinnitus is easy to fix. But even if it's not, there are plenty of nondrug ways to quiet the ringing in your ears.

- Ask your doctor or pharmacist if any of your prescription or over-the-counter medications can cause ringing in the ears. Examples include antibiotics, diuretics or water pills like furosemide (Lasix), antidepressants like amitriptyline (Elavil,) nonsteroidal anti-inflammatory drugs like ibuprofen (Motrin), and even high doses of aspirin. A word of caution — never stop taking a drug your doctor prescribed without his approval.
- Try eliminating ingredients that may make tinnitus worse, such as caffeine, alcohol, salt, and artificial sweeteners. Eliminate them one at time to narrow down the possible culprits.
- Get your hearing checked, and get a hearing aid if you need one. This might stop your brain from filling in the gaps in your hearing with that ringing sound.

- Eat more foods rich in vitamin B12. A small study from Israel found that people with tinnitus and hearing loss were more likely to be deficient in this vitamin. Twelve people who improved their B12 levels saw improvements in their tinnitus, too. If you are an older adult, you may not be able to absorb enough B12 from your food to help. In that case, ask your doctor about checking your vitamin B12 levels to see if you should take supplements.
- Nicotine can make tinnitus worse. Quit smoking.
- Deficiencies in zinc, vitamin D, or coenzyme Q10 can affect your hearing. Enjoy more foods that are rich in these nutrients such as beef or peanut butter for zinc, fish or fortified milk for vitamin D, and fish for coenzyme Q10. Ask your doctor if you need supplements for any of these nutrients.
- Magnesium can help fight hearing loss and tamp down tinnitus. Make sure you are not short on magnesium. Enjoy more magnesium-rich foods like bran cereal, black beans, almonds, and leafy greens like spinach.
- Experiment with masking. See if you can drown out the annoying sounds. Tune a radio between stations so it plays static, or run a fan. Humidifiers, white noise machines, and nature sound machines are also good to try.
- Loud noise makes tinnitus worse. Avoid or limit your exposure to loud sounds, and be ready to whip out your earplugs at a moment's notice to protect your ears.
- Stress aggravates tinnitus. Reduce or eliminate some of the stress in your life. Try relaxation techniques like deep breathing, meditation, or yoga.

Folk remedy tackles tinnitus

Ginkgo biloba is commonly used to treat poor blood flow. So unsurprisingly, it may help tinnitus by increasing blood circulation to your inner ear. This herb may also fend off free radicals, unstable and dangerous molecules that can cause ear damage.

That's not all. Improved blood flow throughout your body may help warm up cold hands and feet caused by poor circulation. If your brain gets more blood, it could sharpen your thinking and help you ward off mild cognitive impairment. Talk to your doctor before trying ginkgo, as it may interact with some medications.

Eat fish for two-way protection

Don't wait until you go to the beach to enjoy seafood. Start eating fish regularly today, and you may lower your odds of hearing loss. Discover how much fish you need to eat, and how your hearing may be connected to your heart.

Australian researchers examined the diets and hearing of nearly 3,000 people age 50 and older. They repeated these exams after five years, and then again 10 years later. The researchers discovered that people who ate two or more servings of fish each week had a 42 percent lower risk of hearing loss than people who ate one serving or less. What's more, a higher intake of the omega-3 fatty acids commonly found in fish was also linked to a drop in the risk of hearing loss.

In fact, the researchers think those omega-3 fatty acids may be why seafood seems to protect your hearing. Animal research suggests your cochlea, a spiral shaped chamber in your inner ear, needs a constant and adequate supply of blood to maintain your hearing.

If heart and blood vessel disease develops as you age, narrowing of the arteries may gradually restrict the blood supply to your cochlea until it begins to suffer damage and function poorly. That poor functioning can lead to hearing loss.

But omega-3 fatty acids from fish can help prevent heart disease by lowering cholesterol and triglycerides, fighting inflammation, and lowering your risk of blood clots. Preventing heart disease and narrowing of the arteries keeps the blood supply to your cochlea flowing, so hearing loss is less likely to occur.

To add fish rich in omega-3 fatty acids to your diet, choose fresh, frozen, or canned salmon, herring, rainbow trout, canned sardines, and light canned tuna. But remember, all fish are not equally safe and healthy to eat, so be sure to take the precautions outlined in "4 things you should know before eating fish" in the *Rheumatoid arthritis* chapter.

Safeguard your ears from cellphone danger

A small Austrian study of cellphone users suggests that people who have used a cellphone for four years or more may have a higher risk of tinnitus than people who have not. More research is needed, but meanwhile, play it safe. Alternate between ears, use your speakerphone, or try a headset or hands-free device.

Heart disease

Sweet way to stave off heart disease

On Valentine's Day, chocolate and hearts make a classic combination. But they may be linked the whole year through. Experts say eating more chocolate could lower your risk of heart disease.

What chocolate can do for you. In an analysis of seven previous studies, researchers found that people who ate the most chocolate:

- reduced their risk of heart disease by 37 percent compared to those who ate the least.
- lowered their risk of stroke by 29 percent.

All forms of chocolate, including chocolate bars, drinks, and cookies, counted in the studies. No distinction was made between dark or milk chocolate. Follow-up ranged from eight to 16 years.

How chocolate helps your heart. The credit probably goes to the high concentration of polyphenols in cocoa products. These antioxidants boost production of the chemical nitric oxide, which helps lower blood pressure and improve blood flow.

Before you overindulge. Don't start gobbling candy bars just yet. This analysis comes with some bittersweet news, too.

Researchers stress that more studies are needed to confirm the link between chocolate and heart health. Keep in mind that these studies were observational studies, so they did not directly test the effects of chocolate. Rather, participants logged their chocolate consumption and researchers kept track of various health outcomes. So something other than chocolate could be at work. There's also the risk that people — especially overweight people with heart disease — underestimated their chocolate intake, skewing the results of these studies.

Remember, many chocolate products are loaded with fat, sugar, and calories. Gorging on chocolate can lead to weight gain and an increased risk of health problems such as high blood pressure, diabetes, and heart disease.

But enjoying an extra chocolate snack now and then shouldn't hurt. It could even be the perfect treat for your heart.

Did you know?

Contrary to popular belief, the darkest chocolate does not always have the most polyphenols. Processing and handling of cocoa seeds changes the antioxidant power of the chocolate. In general, look for dark chocolate that's less processed — no alkalinization — and is closer to its natural form.

Strike down strokes with apples and pears

A Dutch study discovered that eating fruits and vegetables with white flesh — such as apples and pears — helped lower the risk of stroke. People in the 10-year study who ate the most foods in this category reduced their risk of stroke by 52 percent compared to those who ate the least.

Researchers classified foods by color according to their fleshy portion, rather than the skin. That's why apples — whether they had red or green skins — fit in the "white" category. Other white foods included bananas, cauliflower, chicory, cucumber, mushrooms, garlic, leeks, and onions.

But apples and pears were the most commonly eaten white foods in this study, accounting for 55 percent of the total. Apple juice and applesauce also counted in this group.

What makes these foods so effective? While many are rich in fiber, apples and pears are packed with quercetin, a powerful antioxidant called a flavonol. Previous studies have shown that dietary fiber can lower blood pressure, which helps lower your risk of stroke, and that a high intake of flavonols can cut strokes by 20 percent.

Interestingly, other colorful foods — including green, orange or yellow, and red or purple fruits and vegetables — did not seem to make a difference on stroke risk. But that doesn't mean you should give up on them. They can still help prevent other health conditions.

The study, which included more than 20,000 people, used food frequency questionnaires to determine eating patterns. That means it relied on people accurately logging what they ate. So researchers say that more research is needed to confirm these promising results.

In the meantime, boost your intake of apples and pears. The study found that each 25-gram per day increase in white fruits and veggies lowered the risk of stroke by 9 percent. A medium apple weighs about 182 grams, and a medium pear tips the scales at 178 grams. So just one extra piece of white fruit a day could work wonders.

Amazing tea unclogs arteries

You really can open your cupboard and scrub your arteries clean. Brew a cup of green tea, and you fight the plaque that's in your arteries as well as the plaque on your teeth related to heart disease. That's right, this delicious drink keeps you in tiptop shape both inside and out. Here's how.

Keeps a lid on bad cholesterol. Black tea is fermented, but green tea leaves are not. That means green tea holds on to lots of polyphenols — natural antioxidants that work to keep you healthy.

Researchers decided to review previous studies to see how the antioxidants in green tea help with high cholesterol. In 14 studies, results showed that drinking green tea or consuming green tea extract lowered total cholesterol and LDL — "bad" — cholesterol. Overall, HDL cholesterol levels did not change.

Catechins in green tea may get the credit. This type of polyphenol works to keep cholesterol from being absorbed from the food you eat. Catechins also seem to keep your body from processing cholesterol — similar to the way statin drugs work. So you could say green tea works like a statin you can drink.

Lowers risk of atherosclerosis. Plaque buildup in your mouth leads to gum disease and inflammation, which is related to heart disease. That means keeping your teeth clean is especially important.

Did you know?

Chew on this for heart protection. Xylitol, a sweetener in some sugarless chewing gum, suppresses mouth bacteria. Kill off excess bacteria in your mouth, and you cut down on plaque and the risk of gum disease. Experts have found that people with gum disease are twice as likely to suffer from heart disease as those without it. So chewing xylitol gum such as Trident may actually protect your heart.

What if you could kill damaging bacteria in your mouth just by drinking tea? You can, and it's because of a certain type of polyphenol in green tea called epigallocatechin gallate — EGCG — which stops *Streptococcus mutans* bacteria from growing and developing into plaque on your teeth.

It's best to brew your own green tea rather than get it from a bottle. Food experts reported that many of the store-bought bottled green tea drinks are not great sources of polyphenols. In fact, you would need to drink 20 bottles of some brands to get the same polyphenols you can get from a single cup of brewed green tea.

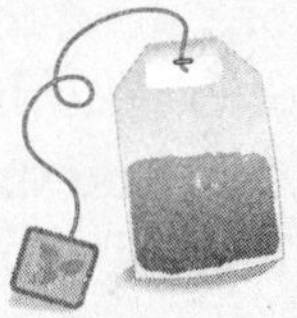

Most of the good-for-you antioxidants from tea seep from the tea leaves and into your beverage within the first minute of brewing. You'll get slightly more antioxidants if you brew for five minutes, but there's no need to wait longer than that — unless you just like really strong tea.

Heal your heart with honey

Mix a spoonful of honey into your green tea, and you'll give your heart a double dose of protection.

Natural honey — the darker the better — is a powerful source of many kinds of antioxidant compounds, including quercetin, flavonoids, and vitamin C. Researchers at the University of Illinois compared various types of honey, and found buckwheat honey has a level of antioxidants as high as many of the most powerful fruits and vegetables.

Honey experts say these natural compounds keep your heart healthy in three ways:

- allows arteries to expand and contract smoothly
- cuts down on excess blood clotting
- lowers the level of LDL — "bad" cholesterol — in your blood

As with any sweet, honey has lots of calories, so you don't want to overdo it. But remember to substitute honey for sugar whenever you can for the health of your heart.

15 heart-healthy foods on a budget

You don't need to break the bank to bring home groceries that will help keep your heart young and strong. Eat cheaply and still eat well when you dig into these 15 healthy foods that won't put a dent in your wallet.

Pick foods from this category	... like these cheap choices	... for these heart benefits
whole grains	brown rice, old-fashioned oats, whole-grain bread	fiber, protein, B vitamins
low-fat dairy	nonfat Greek yogurt	calcium, protein, low in calories
colorful fruits	oranges, pears, apples	fiber, potassium, vitamin C, low in calories
powerhouse vegetables	broccoli, sweet potatoes, spinach	fiber, potassium, numerous vitamins, low in calories
seafood	canned salmon	omega-3 fatty acids, protein
beverages	green tea	numerous antioxidants
meat substitutes	fat-free refried beans, dried lentils, egg substitute	low-fat protein

3 great reasons to eat apricots

The word "apricot" means "precious" in Latin, because these little gems ripen so early in the season. You'll call apricots precious, as well, when you learn what they can do for your health.

Fend off heart disease. Apricots are jam-packed with potassium, a key mineral that helps balance out extra salt in your diet and neutralize its heart-damaging effects. In fact, research found that people who eat too much sodium and too little potassium are more than twice as likely to die of a heart attack compared with people who eat about the same amounts of each.

Start your morning with a cup of sliced fresh apricots, and you're getting a hefty 427 milligrams (mg) of potassium, a big part of what you'll need for the day. If you prefer, grab a handful of dried apricots for a snack, and you get a whopping 650 mg of potassium.

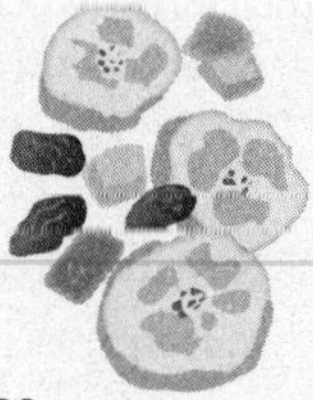

Dried fruits can be just as healthful as their fresh versions, experts say.

"Dried fruits are great sources of total and soluble fiber in the diet," says Dr. Daniel D. Gallaher of the University of Minnesota. "Just as fresh fruit, they have low Glycemic Index values and can play an important role in preventing different aspects of metabolic diseases."

Gallaher and other food scientists want to give traditional dried fruits — among the top sources of potassium and containing a variety of antioxidants, vitamins, and minerals — equal billing with fresh fruits in nutrition recommendations.

That's because they are fairly cheap, easy to store and transport, and don't spoil quickly.

Stamp out stroke risk. Getting lots of potassium may also cut your risk of stroke. That's what researchers found when they analyzed data on potassium and heart disease from 11 different studies. People who got at least 1,640 mg of potassium a day — less than the daily recommended amount of 2,600 mg for women and 3,400 mg for men — had a 21 percent lower risk of stroke than people who got less. This may be due to the fact that potassium lowers blood pressure, or maybe because it also slows down the development of atherosclerosis by preventing artery walls from thickening.

Watch your weight without dieting. Whether you enjoy apricots fresh or dried, even one sweet and juicy serving is just the ticket to help control your weight. The 3 grams of fiber in a cup of fresh slices helps fill you up and keep you from snacking on more calorie-dense goodies. And experts say people who eat dried fruit regularly — as little as 1/8 cup a day — tend to weigh less and have smaller waistlines. Be sure your dried apricots have no added sugar, and they'll pack just 67 calories per 1-ounce serving.

Eat like the ancients for super health

Seems like the more researchers look for new ways to make food healthy, the more they find that old ways are best for your body. Check out these foods from the Bible, now proven by science to prevent disease, slow aging, and even reverse the symptoms of potentially deadly conditions.

honey	apples	cumin
vinegar	figs	mustard
olive oil	dates	wheat
fish	almonds	barley
grape juice	pomegranates	beans
milk	cinnamon	lentils
cheese	garlic	onions

Change your oil for a healthy body

Olive oil is mentioned in the Bible over 100 times — and for good reason. Science has discovered that this ancient remedy is loaded with a compound that protects your heart, lowers your cholesterol, fights cancer, and more. It's called oleocanthal, and it's abundant in extra virgin olive oil. What's more, this tasty Mediterranean staple has other natural chemicals that protect your health.

Stops stroke. Researchers tested whether olive oil might protect older folks who never had a stroke. They surveyed nearly 8,000 people age 65 and older to find out how much olive oil they used for cooking, in salad dressing, and on bread. They also tested blood levels of oleic acid, an important omega-9 fatty acid in olive oil. Five years later, the researchers checked to see how many people in the group had suffered strokes.

Turns out people who ate the most olive oil had a 41 percent lower risk of stroke than those who never ate olive oil. Having a high blood level of oleic acid also seemed to offer protection, with those in the highest group enjoying a 73 percent lower risk of stroke.

Hampers heart disease. The natural chemicals in olive oil also may help prevent heart disease by blocking inflammation. Researchers found that people with high blood pressure who ate food cooked with olive oil were 48 percent less likely to develop heart disease. Triglycerides, total cholesterol, and "bad" LDL cholesterol were all lower in people who ate olive oil.

Olive oil protects your heart for a couple of reasons. The oleocanthal in it works like a nonsteroidal anti-inflammatory drug that reduces the risk of cardiovascular disease. And its plant sterols limit your body's ability to absorb cholesterol, which helps keep your arteries clean.

Inhibits inflammation. Along with heart disease, inflammation plays a role in other health problems including arthritis, Alzheimer's disease, and some cancers.

- Research on animals shows oleocanthal in olive oil may protect nerve cells in your brain from toxic proteins associated with Alzheimer's disease. In addition, olive oil's healthy fats protect brain cells against age-related damage.
- Oleocanthal also gets credit for blocking tumor growth in certain cancers, including those found in the breast, colon, lung, and prostate. Experts are checking on links between the anti-inflammatory powers of olive oil and cell apoptosis — the self-destruction of a cancer cell.
- Anti-inflammatory compounds in olive oil, including oleocanthal, have also been shown to cut inflammation that can damage joints in people with rheumatoid arthritis. It also may work to protect your joints if you have osteoarthritis.

Get fish oil straight from the fish

Some 20 percent of seniors in the United States take fish oil supplements to protect their hearts. If you count yourself among them, you may want to think twice. Experts aren't so sure that these pills provide many health benefits. Even worse, if you don't already have heart problems, they may do more harm than good. A study of more than 415,000 people found that healthy people who regularly took fish oil supplements were more likely to have a stroke or atrial fibrillation.

The good news? Eating fish doesn't seem to have the same drawbacks. Research suggests that getting omega-3 fatty acids straight from the source could be a safer way to keep your heart healthy.

A study found that older women who ate at least five servings a week of baked or broiled fish — but not fried fish — were 30 percent less likely to have heart failure than those who rarely ate it.

Women got the strongest protection from eating dark fish like salmon, mackerel, or bluefish, all of which have high levels of healthy omega-3 fatty acids. In contrast, eating tuna or white fish like sole, snapper, or cod provided less protection.

Most people eat around 20 times more omega-6 fatty acids than omega-3s. That's bad news, because eating too much omega-6 can increase inflammation in your body and make it harder for you to use omega-3 fatty acids. You'll find omega-6s in corn-fed beef and some vegetable oils, like soybean and safflower.

Did you know?

Can't seem to get your cholesterol to go down, even if you don't eat a lot of butter, red meat, and tropical oils like coconut and palm oil? It may have nothing to do with those foods. The hidden cause of your high cholesterol may be a genetic disorder called familial hypercholesterolemia (FH).

This condition prevents the body from removing LDL cholesterol from the bloodstream, which can lead to atherosclerosis and heart attacks at an early age.

Still, you may want to consider a low-carb diet if you have FH. The reason? Many people with this condition who develop coronary heart disease also show risk factors for metabolic syndrome — that's high blood sugar, high blood pressure, and extra body fat around the waist.

Experts say people can manage metabolic syndrome with a low-carb diet. That's because this disorder is associated with carbohydrate intolerance, which occurs when the body has a hard time digesting sugars and starches. Talk to your doctor about making the switch from high-carb foods like breads, potatoes, and sweets to fish, leafy greens, and nuts.

Follow the recommendations of the American Heart Association and aim for two servings of fish a week. To avoid the extra calories that come with frying, it's best to bake, broil, or steam it.

Antioxidant spices cut high-fat dangers

Add certain spices to your next high-fat meal, and maybe you can enjoy that treat just a little bit more.

Researchers tested how spices high in antioxidants might cut the negative effects of eating fat — normally a high-fat meal causes your triglycerides, a dangerous type of fat, to go up. If your triglycerides go too high, too often, you're at a greater risk of heart disease.

For the study, men ate a meal containing 49 grams of fat — coconut chicken, white rice, cheese bread, and a cookie. A week later, they ate the same meal with 2 tablespoons of antioxidant-rich spices added — rosemary, oregano, turmeric, black pepper, cloves, garlic powder, paprika, ginger, and cinnamon.

After each meal, the researchers tested the men's blood every 30 minutes to see how high their triglycerides were rising. When they ate the spicy meal, their triglyceride response was 30 percent lower than when they ate the bland meal. Overall, the researchers took the test results as evidence that certain spices may override the negative effects of fatty food.

Just don't go whole-hog with fried foods, thinking a pinch of curry will protect you. Aim to eat right at most meals, with an occasional indulgence.

Top 12 anti-aging foods

Pick foods and spices that contain lots of antioxidants to supercharge your immune system and disease-proof your body. These easy-to-find, inexpensive choices are loaded with nutrients that fend off heart disease, cancer, premature aging, and much more.

In fact, research found that women who ate an antioxidant-rich diet had a lower risk of stroke, no matter their health history.

Top antioxidant-rich foods and spices	
acai	cloves
black raspberries	oregano
pecans	rosemary
elderberries	thyme
walnuts	cinnamon
golden raisins	turmeric

Protect your arteries with pecans

Here's a nutty way to keep your arteries young, fit, and flexible — eat more pecans.

Not only do they lower your cholesterol, these nuts also prevent LDL cholesterol — the bad kind — from becoming oxidized. That's good because once it's oxidized, it's more likely to build up in your arteries and lead to atherosclerosis.

> Erectile dysfunction (ED) and heart problems may both be caused by poorly functioning blood vessels. Doctors often miss this important connection, so let your physician know your ED could be a sign of a potential heart attack before it happens.

What gives pecans such power? They are loaded with antioxidants, including a form of vitamin E called gamma-tocopherol, the flavonoid catechin, and proanthocyanidins. Even though pecans are also high in fat, this army of antioxidants seems to counteract fat's negative effects.

In a Loma Linda University study, 16 people ate three different test meals with a one-week washout period between each one. The meals consisted of 90 grams, or about 3 ounces, of whole pecans plus water, the same amount of pecans blended with water, and a control meal with no pecans. Here's what happened.

- Eight hours after eating the pecan meals, blood concentrations of gamma-tocopherol doubled.
- While cholesterol levels did not change after the pecan meals, oxidized LDL cholesterol decreased by 30 percent after two hours, 33 percent after three hours, and 26 percent after eight hours.

Researchers aren't sure exactly how pecans and other nuts help protect your heart. But it's likely that gamma-tocopherol and catechin — or possibly both of them working in tandem — provide key antioxidant benefits.

Just a few handfuls of pecans a day should do the trick. You can snack on pecans between meals or sprinkle them into salads for added crunch. Pecans also go great in homemade pies, cakes, and cookies.

Savory spiced pecans

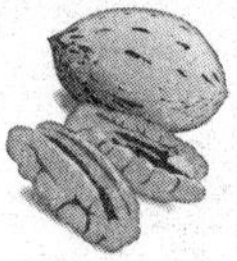

1 1/2 teaspoons salt
1/2 teaspoon cayenne pepper or curry powder
3/4 teaspoon black pepper
2 teaspoons cinnamon
2 tablespoons brown sugar
4 cups pecan halves
3 tablespoons butter

Preheat oven to 350 degrees Fahrenheit. Mix spices and sugar in a bowl. Spread pecan halves in a large frying pan and heat on low for 10 minutes, stirring occasionally.

Remove pecans from pan. Add butter to the pan and melt. Add warm pecans to melted butter and stir, coating the nuts in butter. Add spice mixture to nuts and toss. Spread nuts on a baking sheet, and toast in the oven for up to five minutes. Cool and store in an airtight container for up to three days.

Easy, cheesy way to protect your heart

To get you to smile, a photographer might tell you to say "cheese." Here's something else worth smiling about — eating cheese may help prevent heart disease.

> As an antioxidant, vitamin K2 is 15 times more powerful than K1.

The secret is vitamin K2, a form of vitamin K found in cheese. If you're not familiar with vitamin K, here's some background on its two main forms — K1 and K2.

- K1, or phylloquinone, is found mostly in green leafy vegetables like lettuce, broccoli, spinach, kale, and Swiss chard. This more common form of vitamin K is also found in plant oils like canola and soybean.
- K2, or menaquinone, is found in fermented food products like cheese and natto, a fermented soybean dish. It can also be found in milk, butter, cottage cheese, and egg yolk. To complicate matters, menaquinones are further classified by their number of side chains. The longer the chain, the longer the half-life in the body, and the more useful it is. So MK-4, the form found in meat and eggs, does not last as long as MK-7. The higher forms of vitamin K2 — MK-7, MK-8, and MK-9 — are the types found in fermented cheese.

Here's what two studies out of the Netherlands found about vitamin K2 and heart disease.

- Data on more than 16,000 women showed that every 10-microgram increase in vitamin K2 led to a 9-percent reduction in the risk of developing heart disease. So more cheese could mean less risk. Results were especially strong for the higher forms of vitamin K2 — MK-7, MK-8, and MK-9. Vitamin K1, however, had no effect on heart disease risk.

- In the earlier Rotterdam Study, a high intake of vitamin K2 reduced the risk of heart disease by 41 percent. It worked by preventing arteries from becoming calcified, or hardened by calcium deposits. A medium or high intake of vitamin K2 reduced the risk of severe aortic calcification by 29 percent and 52 percent, respectively.

> You'll eat lots of Emmental cheese when you enjoy classic Swiss fondue.

Although high in fat and salt, cheese does not seem to increase the risk of heart disease. In fact, researchers speculate that high cheese consumption in France and Mediterranean countries could contribute to their lower rates of heart disease.

Adding low-fat cheese and curds to your diet could help safeguard your heart. Which cheeses should you choose? Japanese researchers determined that Norwegian Jarlsberg and Swiss Emmental have the highest levels of MK-9, followed by Raclette and Comte.

Lowly beans a heart-smart choice

Beans really are good for your heart. Just one serving a day of this cheap, tasty, down-home staple cuts heart attack risk by more than a third, and may also prevent sudden cardiac death.

Head off a heart attack. Researchers out of Harvard wanted to study how beans alone — not including peanuts or other legumes — might protect you from having a second heart attack. So they looked at a group of people who tend to eat a lot of beans — folks in Costa Rica. In particular, researchers studied men who had already survived a heart attack, comparing those who said they almost never ate beans with those who ate them every day.

> Sudden cardiac death results from sudden cardiac arrest, a condition in which the heart suddenly and unexpectedly stops beating. It is not the same as a heart attack, and most people die within minutes.

They found that people who ate beans at least once a day had a 38 percent lower risk of a second heart attack. The researchers were not surprised at these results, since beans contain great heart-smart nutrients such as fiber, folate, minerals like magnesium and potassium, and complex carbohydrates.

Prevent SCD. Beans can also cut the risk of sudden cardiac death (SCD), usually related to heart rhythm problems in people who didn't even know they were sick.

Experts looking at over 88,000 nurses found that women with high levels of magnesium in their blood had a 37 percent lower risk of SCD over the 26-year study. Since magnesium — plentiful in beans — works with other minerals to regulate your heartbeat, it's not surprising that beans can keep your heart beating strong.

Live a long, healthy life. Researchers decided to test how bean eaters around the world — from Japan, Greece, Sweden, and Australia — fared in comparison to those who avoided beans. The research was part of the "Food Habits in Later Life" study, which looked at diets of seniors to see which foods were related to longevity.

The results found that the more legumes people ate, the lower their risk of death. The seven-year study considered common legumes in the various countries — lentils, chickpeas, peas, soy, white beans, and others — all available at any grocer.

Did you know?

"Bad" LDL cholesterol can harden the walls of your arteries and block blood flow. But there's a natural way to rejuvenate your arteries and leave you feeling brand new. White grape juice can raise your "good" HDL cholesterol level. HDL picks up extra cholesterol in your blood and carries it to your liver where it's broken down and removed from your body.

Get triple protection from black beans

All beans are good for your heart and your health, but one phenomenal bean is your best bet when it comes to heart disease, diabetes, and stroke protection. It's the black bean, and it can help safeguard your health because of four components.

Fiber. Black beans are bursting with fiber, which research shows can cut your risk of heart-related death by:

- improving blood fat levels.
- enhancing insulin resistance.
- lowering blood pressure.

With 15 grams per cup, black beans outpace kidney beans, garbanzo beans, and lima beans when it comes to fiber content.

Antioxidants. The antioxidants in black beans slow the process of LDL cholesterol building up in and hardening your arteries, a condition called atherosclerosis that brings on blood flow problems. Fortunately, it's easy to get more antioxidant-rich black beans in your diet. You can blend them into your smoothies for a healthy breakfast, or mash them up with some cooked onion and garlic for a healthy alternative to mashed potatoes.

Magnesium. You need this mineral to keep your heart pumping and blood flowing smoothly. Black beans are a great source, and a cup gives you roughly 30 percent of your daily requirement.

In addition, a study found that people who consumed the most magnesium from foods and supplements were about half as likely to develop diabetes in the next 20 years as those not getting as much.

Folate. Finally, you'll get a heaping helping of folate in every serving of black beans. This important B vitamin, along with vitamin B6, lowers the level of artery-damaging homocysteine in your body. Researchers in Japan who looked at the diets of nearly

59,000 people between the ages of 40 and 79 found that women who ate the most folate and vitamin B6 were less likely to die of stroke or heart disease during the 14-year study. Men cut their risk of dying from heart failure.

Black bean brownies

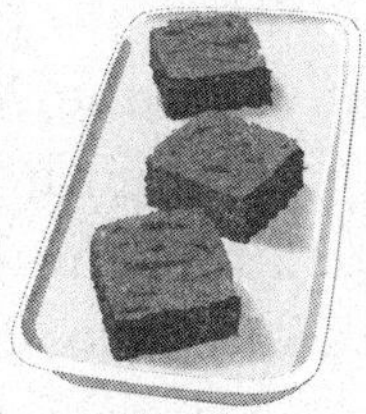

Beans are the perfect meat substitute, letting you skip artery-clogging saturated fat while still getting essential amino acids and other important nutrients. They can help you:

- cut your food budget since beans are so inexpensive.
- make healthier meals since they're chock-full of vitamins and minerals.
- keep your waistline slim since the soluble fiber in beans controls belly fat.

Here's a surprising way to substitute black beans for all the fat in your next batch of brownies.

Drain a 15 1/2-ounce can of black beans. Puree until smooth in a blender or food processor. Stir the beans into your dry brownie mix along with about 4 tablespoons of water — enough to get a typical brownie consistency. Omit the eggs, oil, and other ingredients called for on the box.

You may need to bake these brownies a bit longer than usual. But they taste great and are so good for you.

Fatty fish fights PAD

Some ordinary aches and pains may not be simple symptoms of aging. They could be warning signs of a more serious problem you shouldn't ignore. Talk to your doctor if you experience:

- muscle cramps after climbing stairs.
- numbness in your legs.
- difficulty walking.

In addition, beware of some more specific symptoms like shiny skin on your legs, coldness in one leg or foot, or a change in the color of your legs. These are all signs that the arteries in your legs might be dangerously clogged with fatty deposits, a condition called peripheral artery disease (PAD).

It's a fairly common disease, affecting up to12 million Americans, but perhaps its greatest danger is that it increases your risk of heart attack or stroke. Your doctor will talk to you about exercise, diet, and medication to control PAD, but there's one easy initiative you can take on your own — eat fish more often.

Fatty fish is a great source of vitamin D, and researchers found a link between vitamin D levels and risk of developing peripheral artery disease.

In a study out of Albert Einstein College of Medicine, people with the highest levels of vitamin D in their blood had a much lower risk of PAD than people with the lowest vitamin D levels. When the scientists adjusted their results, taking into account factors like age and other health problems, they found PAD was 64 percent more common among people with the lowest blood levels of vitamin D. Experts are still investigating several reasons behind this relationship.

You can get a good serving of vitamin D from fatty fish like salmon or bluefin tuna, especially if it's caught in the wild, fortified dairy foods, and some fish oil supplements like cod liver oil. Your body also makes vitamin D — "the sunshine vitamin" — when you spend time in the sun, so don't hide indoors. Grab a friend and a fishing pole, get outside on a sunny day, and catch yourself a serving of artery protection.

> The recommended amounts of vitamin D are 600 international units (IU) or 15 micrograms (mcg) for people age 51 to 70 and 800 IU or 20 mcg for anyone age 71 or older.

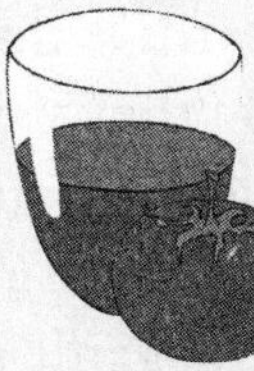

You won't believe this, but it's true. Tomato juice could lower your cholesterol painlessly. It may even prevent heart attacks.

A study of people with diabetes found that just two glasses of this drink a day could boost LDL cholesterol's resistance to oxidation. That's important because oxidized LDL cholesterol can lead to heart attacks. But lycopene, the pigment in tomatoes that gives them their red color, may help prevent this dangerous cholesterol from forming.

Natural 'pill' wards off heart attack and stroke

Some foods and spices have the reputation of working like medicine. That's the case with garlic, traditionally called everything from "nectar of the gods" to "stinking rose." That pungent smell, which gets your attention right away, is due to the very components that make garlic good for you — sulfur compounds like allicin and hydrogen sulfide.

Researchers say that adding garlic supplements to your daily routine or eating plenty of this superfood could help clogged arteries virtually disappear and prevent heart disease.

Say "sayonara" to high cholesterol. Sulfur-containing compounds in garlic may help keep blood lipids in balance. Studies show eating garlic can bring down total cholesterol by up to 12 percent, and it also lowers bad LDL cholesterol and triglycerides.

Give heart attacks the heave-ho. Researchers tested giving Allicor, a brand of powdered-garlic supplement, to people with heart disease, comparing them with people who took a placebo. Each group took one pill twice a day for a year, with the Allicor group taking 150 milligrams of garlic powder.

The researchers then tallied how many heart attacks and cases of sudden cardiac death had occurred in the folks in the study, and how likely they were to have these problems within 10 years. Men being studied were much less likely — one-and-a-half times less likely — to have a heart attack or sudden cardiac death if they had been taking garlic supplements. Women were also safer after taking garlic compared with the placebo, but the difference was less striking than in men. Researchers think that may simply be due to how few women were in the study.

Stop a stroke in its tracks. Experts say aged garlic extract is an especially potent antioxidant, protecting cells in artery walls and preventing blood platelets from clumping together and forming clots. Other studies say this herbal remedy may reduce the buildup of arterial plaque, which can help ward off life-threatening strokes.

Enjoy your garlic-laden pasta dishes knowing your heart enjoys the treat as much as you do. But stay away from garlic supplements if you take blood thinners. They can interact with these drugs and increase your risk of bleeding.

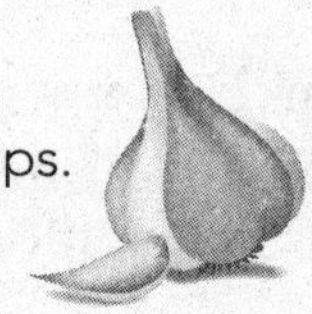

Handle fresh garlic with care to get more of its heart-healthy benefits. Remember these two tips.

- Use garlic in as fresh a form as possible. That means you should try to slice or crush the cloves just before you use them so they hold on to the most hydrogen sulfide. This volatile compound works as a chemical messenger in your body, relaxing blood vessels to improve blood flow. Processing garlic or even crushing it, then letting it dry for a few days, reduces the amount of hydrogen sulfide.
- If you must cook the garlic, crush it first. This process allows the allicin in garlic to do a better job of preventing blood clots. But don't cook it for any longer than necessary.

Herbal supplement dangers

Herbal supplements may seem like natural choices to deal with a health problem. But some of the most popular herbs should never be taken with prescription drugs. Check out this lifesaving list, and talk to your doctor or pharmacist about any potential interactions.

Supplement	Drug class to avoid	Possible risk
echinacea	fibrates, statins, niacin arrhythmia drugs like amiodarone (Cordarone)	liver damage EKG changes
fish oil	blood thinners	bleeding
garlic pills	aspirin, warfarin (Coumadin), clopidogrel (Plavix), heparin	bleeding
ginkgo biloba	aspirin, warfarin (Coumadin)	bleeding
ginseng	digoxin (Lanoxin) warfarin (Coumadin	interferes with blood tests reduces warfarin's effectiveness
hawthorn	nitrates, calcium-channel blockers, digoxin (Lanoxin)	increases potency, likelihood of side effects
red yeast rice	blood thinners statins	bleeding additive effect
saw palmetto	aspirin, clopidogrel (Plavix), warfarin (Coumadin)	bleeding
St. John's wort	clopidogrel (Plavix) digoxin (Lanoxin) warfarin (Coumadin)	bleeding lowers blood levels of digoxin reduces warfarin's effectiveness

Send heart attack risk to a watery grave

Picking water as your beverage of choice may cut your chances of dying of a heart attack in half. That's what California researchers found when they surveyed more than 20,000 men and women about their drinking habits.

The researchers asked people to list how much water or other drinks — fruit juice, milk, alcohol, and caffeinated beverages — they consumed every day. Women who drank more than five 8-ounce glasses of water daily were 41 percent less likely to die from a heart attack during the next six years than those who drank two glasses or less. Among men, drinking five glasses of water cut their risk of heart attack death by 54 percent.

The researchers think not drinking enough water and becoming dehydratedd can raise the viscosity, or thickness, of your blood, and possibly lead to blood clots and heart attack. They even suggest that the well-known higher risk of having a heart attack in the early morning might be due to not drinking overnight.

Surprisingly, people who drank lots of beverages other than water actually seemed to raise their risk of dying from a heart attack. The reason may be that during digestion your body has to work hard to dilute other drinks when consumed in large volumes. To get the job done, water moves from your blood into your digestive system, thickening your blood even more.

So go with a drink that's calorie-free, refreshing, and the best beverage for your heart.

Sip your way to wide-open arteries

When you need a change from drinking water, pour a glass of orange juice to keep your blood vessels in tiptop shape.

HEALTH ALERT!

Beware of these six beverages you should never drink when taking certain medications.

- Orange juice. Natural compounds in OJ block your body's ability to absorb certain beta blockers, some antibiotics, and other drugs.
- Apple juice. Studies show apple juice may interact with the same drugs as orange juice.
- Grapefruit juice. A substance in grapefruit juice, called naringin, can cause certain drugs, including some statins and blood pressure drugs, to build up to toxic levels in your body.
- Cranberry juice. Avoid drinking too much of this while taking blood thinners like warfarin (Coumadin). Cranberry juice can increase the anticlotting effects and cause a hemorrhage.
- Milk. Don't take antibiotics, including doxycycline and ciprofloxacin (Cipro), or the thyroid drug levothyroxine (Synthroid) with calcium-rich dairy products.
- Tea or coffee. Anti-anxiety drugs like diazepam (Valium) and antibiotics such as ciprofloxacin can increase the effects of caffeine, making you more excited and nervous.

Reduces artery inflammation. Researchers in California found taking supplements of vitamin C can cut the level of C-reactive protein (CRP) in your blood. This natural chemical is an indicator of inflammation in your body and a predictor of heart disease and diabetes. People in the study took either 1,000 milligrams of vitamin C, 800 international units of vitamin E, or a placebo every day.

After two months of taking vitamin C, people whose CRP levels had been high at the start had close to a 17 percent decrease in CRP. Those who started with lower, less-dangerous CRP levels did not show such an improvement, and those who took either vitamin E or a placebo also did not get the benefit.

Orange juice is a great source of vitamin C. A cup of fresh juice boasts 124 milligrams of vitamin C, more than you need in a day but far less than you can get from supplements.

Raises "good" cholesterol. A small study found that people with high cholesterol who drank 3 cups of orange juice daily had lower LDL — "bad" cholesterol — and higher HDL — "good" cholesterol — after 60 days. Even those who started the study with cholesterol levels in the normal, healthy range had improved HDL levels after drinking orange juice.

Experts say antioxidant vitamins, including vitamin C, help your heart by making blood vessels more elastic so they expand and contract easier. This change can improve your body's ability to process blood sugar and lipids and control blood pressure.

Widens arteries to cut blood pressure. A natural antioxidant compound in orange juice, hesperidin, gets credit for lowering high blood pressure in a group of healthy men who drank 2 cups a day. After four weeks, their diastolic blood pressure — the bottom number in the reading — was 5.5 points lower than at the start.

Combats memory loss, depression, and more. This same orange juice study also found that people who enjoy their OJ had higher levels of nitric oxide (NO) in their blood. A natural compound made by cells in the walls of your blood vessels, NO opens up blood vessels to increase blood flow to your brain. Better blood flow can give a boost to your mood and battle memory loss, tinnitus, and dizziness.

Pile on the peppers to head off stroke

You are what you eat — especially when it comes to water-soluble vitamins like vitamin C. This powerhouse antioxidant is not stored in your body long-term, so you have to get it from the food you

HEALTH ALERT!

The next time you donate blood, pay attention to your type. If you're a woman with type B or AB blood or a man with type AB blood, you have a greater risk of stroke than people with type O blood. That's what researchers found when they looked at people's stroke risk over a few decades. People with type AB blood had an especially high risk — 26 percent higher than those with type O.

The researchers don't know how blood type might be related to stroke, but previous studies have found that people with type B blood tend to have higher cholesterol levels and blood pressure.

Of course, you can't change your blood type, but knowing you're at risk may encourage you to make healthy changes. Your healthcare provider may soon be able to type your blood with a new quick and cheap "dipstick" test.

eat every day. In fact, a quick blood test can give scientists a clue about what you've been eating lately. Going heavy on the oranges and bell peppers? Lots of vitamin C will show up in your blood. This type of eating plan might help you avoid having a stroke.

Researchers checked this idea by testing blood samples from almost 21,000 middle-aged and older people in England. They divided the participants into five groups based on blood levels of vitamin C. Then they kept tabs on as many people as they could, tracking how many had a stroke over the next nine years. Turns out people with the most vitamin C in their blood had a 42 percent lower risk of stroke than those with the least vitamin C.

You can start the day with a glass of vitamin C–rich orange juice or a tasty grapefruit half, but you may want other options for the rest of the day. Pick peppers, the true heavy hitters when it comes to vitamin C content. A cup of uncooked sweet red peppers has 175 milligrams of vitamin C — more than you can get from a cup of orange juice.

Other forms of peppers, including green bell peppers and hot chili peppers, either raw or cooked, also boast lots of vitamin C. So slice them on your salad, toss them into your stir-fry, and load up your tacos with these tasty stroke busters.

High blood pressure

5 foods you should never eat

The American Heart Association recommends limiting your sodium intake to 1,500 milligrams (mg) a day. That's especially important if you have high blood pressure, or hypertension, since too much salt can damage your heart and arteries and raise your blood pressure.

You can cut back by tossing your salt shaker and cooking meals from scratch rather than relying on processed foods. Avoid these five foods that can bust your low-salt diet, and try out the lower-sodium alternatives.

- Smoked salmon. A 3.5-ounce serving of lox adds about 2,000 mg of sodium to your diet — 33 times as much as the same amount of grilled salmon. Take the time to grill a piece of fresh or frozen salmon, and you're down to just 61 mg of sodium.

> Research shows that people with normal blood pressure may not benefit from a low-salt diet. In fact, eating too little sodium raised the risk of dying from heart disease.

- Packaged meat broth. Whether it's from a can, cube, or envelope, these flavor enhancers are like little salt bombs. A single cube packs 840 mg sodium. Save the pan drippings from your next pot roast instead.
- Powdered gravy. These labor savers do a number on your sodium intake, with 348 mg in a teaspoon of dry gravy mix. It's worth the trouble to make your own gravy so that you can control what goes in the pot.

- Instant pudding. A serving of pudding mix has 340 mg of sodium. Cut back on that number by choosing 8 ounces of low-fat yogurt, with just 125 mg of sodium.
- Processed meat. Skip the bacon and salami, which have salt added at the factory. Roast a chicken and carve it up, and you have sandwich meat for several days — at just 64 mg of sodium in half a chicken breast.

Replace salt with heavenly herbs

Cut down on salt without missing out on taste. Flavor your vegetables, soups, and fish with these seasonings recommended by the American Heart Association.

Fresh or dried herb	Best to season these foods
basil	fish, lean ground meat, stews, salads
chives	salads, vegetables, soups, lean meats
dill	fish sauces, tomatoes, cabbage, carrots, potatoes, lean beef, chicken, fish
rosemary	chicken, lean pork, potatoes, peas, lima beans
sage	lean meats, stews, green beans, tomatoes, lima beans
thyme	lean pork, soups, peas, tomatoes, salads

Keep sodium in check with veggies

About half of U.S. adults regularly take vitamin and mineral pills, spending some $12 billion a year for this nutritional insurance. Besides costing a lot of money, these supplements may actually be bad for your health.

Research shows older women who regularly take nutritional supplements are at slightly higher risk of dying than those who don't take supplements. Researchers followed nearly 39,000 women for 19 years, tracking their supplement use and recording how they fared as they aged. Even a basic multivitamin raised the risk of dying, but iron supplements were the biggest problem, raising risk of death by 3.9 percent over the course of the study. Rely on foods to get the vitamins and minerals you need for better health, including blood pressure control.

In fact, potassium, a critical mineral, can balance out too much sodium in your diet, relaxing artery walls and encouraging the release of nitric oxide to keep blood pressure in check. Most people don't get the recommended amount of potassium, which is 2,600 milligrams (mg) a day for women and 3,400 mg for men.

Consider these powerhouse vegetables, which offer lots and lots of potassium.

- A single baked potato gives you 1,081 mg.
- A cup of lima beans provides 955 mg.
- A cup of cooked spinach gives you 839 mg.
- One sweet potato has 694 mg.
- A cup of cooked winter squash comes in at 644 mg.

Even a simple can of mixed vegetables gets you well on your way to eating more potassium. Besides, high potassium vegetables have many other nutrients to offer, plus they're tasty and safe to eat.

Did you know?

Staying active may help balance out a high-salt diet. Researchers tested how exercise affected blood pressure in a group of adults in China. People in the study ate either 3,000 milligrams (mg) of sodium a day, or an astoundingly high-sodium diet of 18,000 mg a day. Those who exercised the most had a 38 percent lower risk of experiencing a rise in blood pressure when they ate the high-salt diet.

Spice up meals for lower blood pressure

Look to garlic to add pizzazz to your meals and you'll never miss salt. On top of that, study after study shows garlic can lower blood pressure and cholesterol. You can get garlic in several forms — fresh, dried, and even in capsules.

Researchers in Australia wanted to expand what's known about garlic's effects on blood pressure. That's why they tested giving garlic supplements to a group that had not previously been studied — people with uncontrolled high blood pressure.

The people in the study were taking blood pressure drugs, but their systolic blood pressure — the upper number in a blood pressure reading — was still 140 mmHG or higher. For three months, participants took four capsules a day of aged garlic extract or similar-looking sugar pills and continued taking their blood pressure medicine.

At the end of the study, those who took the garlic extract had systolic blood pressure an average of 10.2 mmHG lower than the people who took the sugar pills. The researchers noted that the benefits of garlic were similar to what might be expected from taking blood pressure medication alone.

Sulfur compounds in garlic, including allicin and hydrogen sulfide, take credit for garlic's medicinal effects. In particular, they change how your body uses nitric oxide, allowing blood vessel walls to relax and let blood flow more easily.

Other research has shown garlic can help keep blood lipids in balance, and fight high triglycerides and LDL cholesterol. For more information about garlic and high cholesterol, as well as other heart-related problems, see "Natural 'pill' wards off heart attack and stroke" in the *Heart disease* chapter.

Much research on this spice uses garlic extracts, powders, or supplements to control the amount of compounds people get. Supplements also let you avoid bad breath or body odor from eating raw garlic.

But many experts say eating garlic can be a great way to help you control your blood pressure.

Improve your odds with onions

Aim for onions to keep high blood pressure in check if garlic is too pungent for your taste. Onions contain an antioxidant flavonoid called quercetin, believed to help battle heart disease, dementia, and diabetes. It also may increase your energy level and help your body fight allergies. Not surprisingly, quercetin is also a boon when it comes to battling high blood pressure.

That's what researchers discovered when they studied middle-aged folks who had either prehypertension or stage 1 high blood pressure. With prehypertension, your upper number is between 120 and 129, while your lower number is below 80. Stage 1 high blood pressure means your upper number is between 130 and 139, while the lower number is between 80 and 89. Half the people in the study took 730 milligrams (mg) of a quercetin supplement daily, while the rest took a sugar pill.

After 28 days, the people with high blood pressure who took the quercetin enjoyed an average drop in blood pressure of 7 mmHG systolic — the upper number in a blood pressure reading — and 5 mmHg diastolic. In fact, quercetin supplements were just as effective in lowering blood pressure as other proven lifestyle changes, such as cutting salt from your diet, exercising more, losing excess weight, and cutting back on alcohol. There was no improvement among people with prehypertension.

Take the bite out of a raw onion, but keep its quercetin. Just wrap some chunks of onion in foil and bake at 390 degrees Fahrenheit for five minutes. More than 99 percent of the quercetin is retained by this cooking method, but the flavor won't overwhelm the rest of the food on your plate.

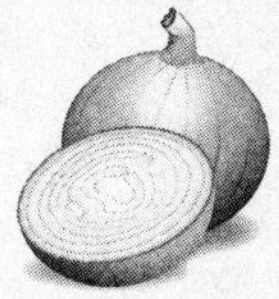

The researchers don't think quercetin's antioxidant powers were at work in lowering blood pressure. Instead, they think quercetin might encourage your body to excrete excess fluids and salt, thus lowering pressure in your arteries.

The average person gets as much as 42 mg of quercetin from a typical day's diet, but you can double that just by eating a single sweet onion. Shop for purple, red, or yellow onions rather than white to get the most quercetin. In general, the darker the color of produce, the more antioxidants it contains. You can also get lots of quercetin from apples, pears, berries, and tea.

Try a DASH of prevention

Want to toss out pills for good and still lower your blood pressure? The Dietary Approaches to Stop Hypertension (DASH) eating plan incorporates tasty, healthy foods to help reduce the sodium in your diet. This age-old solution may be more effective than modern medicine, and can cut your blood pressure by eight to 14 points — more with exercise and weight loss.

Working these foods that fight high blood pressure into your diet is a tasty way to preserve your health.

Helpful components	Great choices
anthocyanins	blueberries, strawberries, raspberries
fiber	cereals with whole grain, like oatmeal and shredded wheat
magnesium	potatoes, halibut, bananas, spinach, kidney beans
potassium	Swiss chard, orange juice, yams, dates, prunes, avocados, cantaloupe, figs, peaches, kale, kiwi, broccoli
nitrates	beet juice, spinach, carrots, lettuce
protein	low-fat yogurt, skim milk
flavonoids	dark chocolate

Sea vegetables help sink high blood pressure

The average person in Japan eats more than 8 pounds of seaweed every year. With these green, brown, and red forms of sea vegetables so common in that country's diet, researchers naturally wanted to find out how seaweed affects health. Turns out seaweed may help keep your blood pressure down.

Researchers in Aichi, Japan, asked a group of parents of preschoolers to record how much seaweed they ate over three days. Then the researchers checked the children's blood pressure and made comparisons with their diets. They found that children who ate more seaweed had lower blood pressure readings. Girls who ate the most seaweed had significantly lower systolic blood pressure, while boys had lower diastolic readings.

Seaweed, similar to many other veggies, is a good source of minerals like calcium, potassium, magnesium, iron, and phosphorus, along with a number of important vitamins. It's low in fat and calories and high in fiber. Some kinds contain up to 47 percent protein.

Did you know?

Wakame is a type of kelp often served in miso soup and salads. Popular in Asian cuisine, this food is now available at your local grocery store or online. That's a good thing because research suggests that wakame can help reduce high blood pressure.

So munch on this tasty sea vegetable and watch your blood pressure drop. Just know that wakame contains a lot of iodine. Your thyroid gland needs this micronutrient to create hormones, but too much of it can lead to thyroid disorders like hyperthyroidism and hypothyroidism.

Because of the harsh growing conditions in the ocean, seaweed also produces other natural plant chemicals. A group called bioactive peptides — short chains of amino acids — is probably responsible for the blood pressure-lowering effect of seaweed. Bioactive peptides in seaweed may behave like ACE inhibitors, drugs that expand blood vessels and regulate fluid in your body to help control blood pressure.

Although the researchers used children in the study, the results suggest the possibility of early life strategies to prevent high blood pressure in adults.

You can add dried seaweed to sandwiches and hummus. Or throw in a couple of sheets next time you're making a smoothie. You can also eat dried seaweed out of the bag for a healthy snack.

Add a piece of dried kombu seaweed to the pot when you cook beans, and they'll turn out more flavorful and have a smoother texture.

Kombu is chock full of glutamates and nucleotides — natural flavor enhancers that bring out the umami, or savory taste, in a dish. Chefs in a professional test kitchen found that adding kombu may even eliminate the need to soak dried beans overnight or brine them for a better texture. You can find kombu at a natural food store or Asian market.

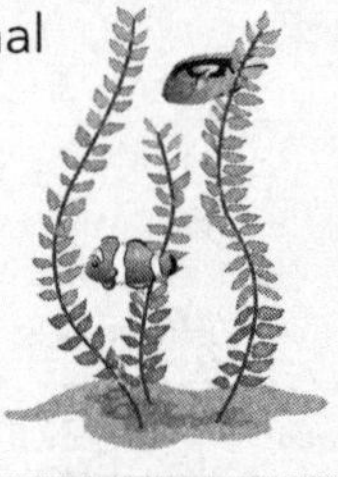

Popular breakfast food lowers blood pressure

When you skip the bacon-and-egg breakfast to keep high blood pressure under control, you still have to find something to eat in the morning. A bowl of whole-grain cereal is your best bet.

Researchers looked at the well-known Physicians' Health Study I to see what foods were common among men with the lowest blood pressure. They found that men who ate whole-grain cereal at least seven times each week had a 20 percent lower risk of developing high blood pressure. Eating cereal fewer times a week also gave some protection, but less with each bowl left uneaten.

Whole-grain cereal has some great ingredients that can battle high blood pressure.

Fiber. Depending on the type of whole-grain cereal you choose, you get a nice serving of insoluble or soluble fiber. Insoluble fiber, found in wheat bran, passes mostly undigested through your intestines. Soluble fiber, plentiful in oats, dissolves in water and may help lower your cholesterol.

Some experts say eating 12 grams of soluble fiber every day may help lower blood pressure. Others point at insoluble fiber as the real blood pressure tamer. When it comes down to it, both types look promising.

Previous research showed eating three servings daily of whole-grain foods led to lower systolic blood pressure. In that study, both insoluble and soluble fiber from wheat and oats seemed to share the same blood pressure-lowering power.

Vitamins and minerals. Many cereals are fortified with the very nutrients your body needs to control blood pressure, like potassium to relax blood vessels and balance out extra sodium in your diet.

Of course, another benefit of eating cereal for breakfast is you avoid unhealthy choices, like glazed doughnuts and sausage biscuits. So consider a heaping helping of rolled oats, shredded wheat, or raisin bran to be a double dose of goodness for lowering blood pressure. Look for the word "whole" before any grains on the label's ingredient list, and opt for a cereal with at least 5 grams of fiber per serving.

Did you know?

Looking for a delicious way to lower blood pressure? Hibiscus tea does it better than even some medications, studies say.

- Researchers found that 2 cups of this strong brew each morning lowered blood pressure as well as a starting dose of captopril, a leading blood-pressure medication.
- Three cups of hibiscus tea every day for six weeks lowered blood pressure in volunteers by seven points, says a study published in *The Journal of Nutrition*.

Scientists think the active ingredient in hibiscus, *H. sabdariffa*, may relax and widen arteries and also act as a diuretic to help your body eliminate extra water and salt.

Although hibiscus is an exotic flower, you don't have to go far to find it. Look for teas with its deliciously tart, cranberry-like flavor in stores and online.

Remarkable grapes to the rescue

Grapes may be the one fruit that can lower both blood pressure and cholesterol. That's because you get both an antioxidant boost and a serving of fiber from grapes. Here's how they help.

Keep blood flowing. Researchers in Spain needed to test the benefits of grapes, so they created a grape supplement to magnify grape ingredients. Named "grape antioxidant dietary fiber" (GADF), this extract was produced from the seeds and skins of grapes.

People with normal cholesterol levels and those with high cholesterol ate the GADF along with their regular meals for 16 weeks. At the end of the study, those who took GADF showed lower blood pressure by up to 5 percent, and both total and LDL cholesterol levels were also down. In fact, among people who had high cholesterol at the start of the study, total cholesterol had dropped by 14 percent and LDL cholesterol by 11 percent after taking the grape extract.

Researcher Jara Perez Jimenez pointed out just how powerful the grape product is.

"The effects appear to be higher than the ones caused by other dietary fibers, such as oat fiber or psyllium, probably due to the combined effect of dietary fiber and antioxidants," Jimenez said. People in the study were getting 5.25 grams of dietary fiber and 1,400 milligrams of polyphenol antioxidants in each GADF serving.

Keep memories strong. And don't forget the juice. Drinking grape juice, along with other fruit and vegetable juices, may also help you avoid Alzheimer's disease (AD) as you age. Researchers in King County, Washington, tracked the diets of older Japanese-American adults over the course of 10 years, noting how many developed dementia. The scientists were interested in finding out why people in Japan had lower rates of AD than Japanese immigrants living in the United States.

The study found that people who drank fruit or vegetable juices more than three times a week were 76 percent less likely to develop this disease than people who drank it less than once a week. The benefit was greatest among people who carry a certain gene that puts them at a higher risk of AD.

Again, the powerful ingredient in fruit juice seems to be its polyphenols — powerful antioxidants abundant in the peels and skins of fruits and vegetables. So drink up your juice to protect your memory, your arteries, and your heart.

Did you know?

If you have high cholesterol, plaque can build up in your arteries and cause them to become too narrow. As a result, your heart has to work extra hard to pump blood throughout your body. That means your blood pressure could go through the roof.

That's where red grapes come in. Scientists found that people with high cholesterol who ate a little more than 3 cups of red grapes daily over two months saw significant improvements in their LDL cholesterol levels. Other research suggests that grape juice may offer similar benefits. A small study found that drinking a little concentrated red grape juice daily for two weeks lowered cholesterol.

Keep numbers down with leafy greens

Leafy greens are an important part of the DASH, or Dietary Approaches to Stop Hypertension, eating plan. Unfortunately, 87 percent of Americans surveyed say they rarely or never eat nutrient-dense greens like Swiss chard or bok choy. Be a part of the other 13 percent by loading your plate with leafy greens. They share four fabulous ingredients to fight the silent killer — high blood pressure.

Folate. This important B vitamin seems to help control blood pressure by interacting with nitric oxide that gets released by cells lining the inside of blood vessels. Nitric oxide helps keep your blood vessels relaxed and flexible, so they can open up and let blood flow smoothly.

Researchers followed more than 150,000 women for eight years to see how folate affected their blood pressure. Study participants in their 30s and 40s cut their risk of high blood pressure almost in half when they got 1,000 micrograms (mcg) of folate daily from both food and supplements.

Besides spinach and other leafy green vegetables, you'll find folate in asparagus, lentils, and pinto beans.

Potassium. When it comes to controlling high blood pressure, potassium packs a powerful punch. It's a key mineral that can balance out too much sodium in your diet and encourage the release of nitric oxide to keep blood pressure in check. An important study of 300 nurses found that potassium can even lower blood pressure that's in the normal range. Spinach, beet greens, turnip greens, baked potatoes, acorn squash, and cantaloupe are great sources of potassium.

Magnesium. Research shows magnesium works to lower blood pressure. In one study, 60 people with high blood pressure took either a magnesium supplement or a placebo. After eight weeks, those taking magnesium had a significant drop in blood pressure. The higher their blood pressure had been at the start, the better results they had.

Magnesium is plentiful in greens like spinach and collards, along with other nutritious foods like avocados and pinto beans.

Calcium. This bone-building mineral keeps your muscles, including your heart, strong and working efficiently. It also helps keep your blood pressure normal. Good green sources of calcium include turnip greens, collard greens, and spinach.

The DASH eating plan also calls for 30 grams of fiber a day. You'll get a good start on that goal with a plate of leafy greens.

Don't get caught in a vicious cycle

High blood pressure and atherosclerosis, or hardening of the arteries, create a vicious cycle, with each one making the other worse.

As blood pressure rises in your arteries, elastic fibers in the walls of the arteries are damaged. That allows artery walls to become more stiff and rigid — and less flexible. When this happens, blood pressure goes up more.

Meanwhile, high pressure in your bloodstream pushes calcium ions in the blood into the artery walls, where they become embedded as plaque and stiffen up the arteries even more. Now artery walls are really stiff and rigid, causing an increase in blood pressure.

And the cycle continues. That's why it's so important to control high blood pressure.

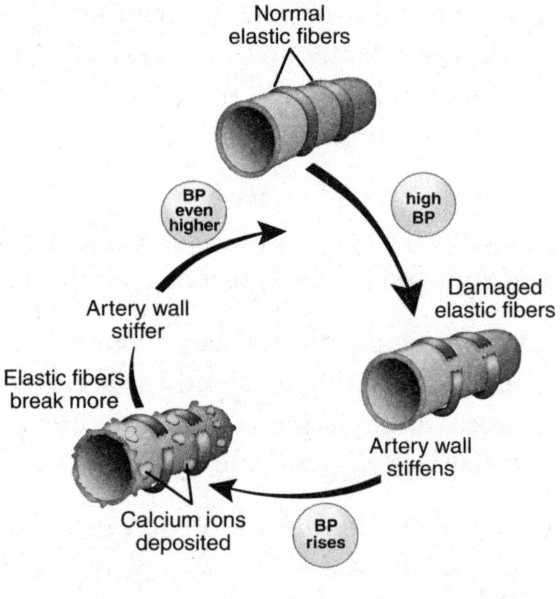

Tap into this powerful remedy

Kiwifruit is the new apple — eat three of these fuzzy gems a day to keep the doctor away.

Researchers in Norway added three kiwis or an apple every day to the diets of adults who had elevated blood pressure readings of around 128/85 mmHG. An ideal blood pressure reading is lower than 120/80 mmHG.

After eight weeks, people who enjoyed the kiwis had systolic blood pressure readings that were 3.6 mmHG lower than those who ate the apples. Systolic pressure is the upper, or first, number in a blood pressure reading.

The researchers think the power in kiwis comes from their high levels of lutein, a carotenoid that works in tandem with the nutrient zeaxanthin to keep your eyes healthy and help prevent vision-stealing cataracts and age-related macular degeneration. Lutein, like beta carotene and other carotenoids, works as an antioxidant to protect cells from damage by free radicals. Antioxidants also help repair damage to artery walls, so clogged arteries can become flexible again and control blood pressure.

Three kiwis give you 279 micrograms (mcg) of lutein and zeaxanthin combined, while an apple provides just 40 mcg of these nutrients. You can also get a hefty serving of lutein from eating leafy greens, like spinach, kale, and collard greens.

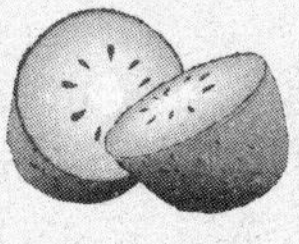

Stop peeling and slicing kiwi, and eat the fruit like they do in Australia and New Zealand. Just slice the top off a kiwi, then scoop out the fruit with a spoon. This easy method lets you eat kiwi anywhere without making a mess. In New Zealand you can even get a "spife," or combination spoon and knife, to toss in a lunch box with your kiwi.

Dig up the secret to lower blood pressure

You can control your blood pressure with colorful spuds — without boosting your weight. Just eat plenty of purple potatoes.

Dieters often cut out potatoes to cut calories, but a study out of the University of Scranton suggests they could be missing out on some serious health benefits.

In the study, 18 overweight or obese people with high blood pressure ate six to eight small purple potatoes with skins twice a day for four weeks. After a month, they lowered their diastolic blood pressure — the bottom number in a blood pressure reading — by an average of 4.3 percent. Their systolic blood pressure, or top number, also dropped an average of 3.5 percent.

> Enjoy blueberries or strawberries with your yogurt or cereal. Research shows a cup of one of these tasty berries, good sources of anthocyanins, may cut your risk of high blood pressure.

The high concentration of antioxidants in purple potatoes, which are rich in anthocyanins and other phytochemicals, could account for their blood pressure-lowering powers. Anthocyanins also give the potatoes their distinctive purple color.

Eating purple potatoes did not cause a spike in blood sugar or fats in the blood. Better yet, none of the participants in the study gained weight. That's probably because they didn't fry the potatoes or slather them in butter or sour cream. Instead, they cooked them in the microwave, a method that helps retain nutrients.

Most of the people in the study were already on blood pressure-lowering medication, but the purple potatoes provided an extra boost. And every bit helps. Remember, keeping your blood pressure and weight under control can help lower your risk of heart disease and stroke.

Eating more purple potatoes may be an easy way to pack a punch against high blood pressure — without packing on the pounds. Look for purple potatoes at your local farmers market or specialty grocery store. Can't find them? Don't worry. Researchers believe red potatoes may also do the trick.

Bag big benefits from a tiny seed

Flaxseed does more than just lower blood pressure. It protects against cancer, too. That's pretty amazing in itself, but doesn't cover all of its abilities. Flaxseed also reduces the risk of stroke, and fights arthritis, stomach disorders, and mental problems.

Fortunately, it's easy to give your meals a little flax appeal. Sprinkle ground flaxseed over your breakfast cereal or blend it into your morning smoothie. Or mix it into lunchtime soups or stews. Delicious! You can also roast whole flaxseeds in a skillet and grind them before adding the flax to your dinner salad.

Out of eggs? No worries. Flax can replace them when you're making muffins, pancakes, cookies, and yeast breads. To replace one egg in your recipe, blend 2 tablespoons of ground flaxseed with 3 tablespoons of cold water. Let the mixture rest for 10 minutes until it has thickened.

To get the longest life out of your flaxseed, store it in the refrigerator or freezer. By keeping ground flaxseed in the fridge, you'll extend its shelf life by one or two months past the expiration date. Freeze it and it will stay fresh up to three months after that date. Whole flaxseed can stay fresh in your freezer for up to a year.

Unexpected help from a snack food

You don't have to go vegetarian to help your heart and lower your blood pressure. But replacing some of the meat in your diet with soy protein may help bring down blood pressure numbers. That's what researchers found when they gave women a daily treat of soy nuts.

In the study, 60 older women took turns eating either the Therapeutic Lifestyle Changes (TLC) diet or a similar plan that replaced some of the diet's protein with soy nuts. The TLC diet is a plan developed by the National Institutes of Health that's low in saturated fat and can help control cholesterol. It relies on lean protein sources like skinless chicken and fatty fish.

When it was their turn to substitute 25 grams of protein in their diet with soy nuts, women in the study ate 1/2 cup of unsalted soy nuts daily. The women could divide up the nuts to eat throughout the day, and they didn't make any other changes in what they ate. The researchers checked up on the women by having them write down everything they ate and testing the level of soy isoflavones in their urine.

After eight weeks, the women with high blood pressure who ate soy nuts had a nearly 10 percent drop in their systolic blood pressure and an almost 7 percent drop in diastolic blood pressure. That's about as much improvement as would be expected from taking drugs to control high blood pressure. Women who started with normal blood pressure also saw lower numbers after eating soy, but not as much of a change.

The secret ingredient in soy nuts is probably genistein, a soy isoflavone or plant estrogen, that can help your blood vessels expand to lower blood pressure. If you don't like soy nuts, you can also get genistein from tofu, soy beans, or soy milk.

Be aware that some research suggests soy isoflavones may contribute to your risk of dementia and help fuel the growth of cancer cells that feed off estrogen. Your best bet is to ask your doctor whether eating soy products is a good choice for you. If he agrees, you can eat foods like soy milk, miso soup, and edamame in moderation.

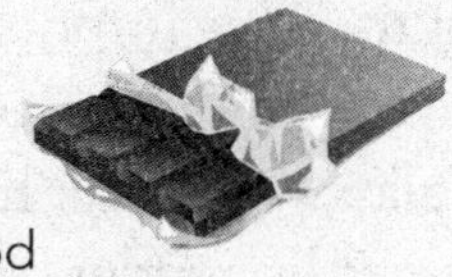

You've read how dark chocolate may cut your risk of stroke and heart disease. Experts say the flavonoids in dark chocolate may also keep your blood pressure down and improve blood flow.

Look for dark chocolate that has a cocoa content of 60 percent or more. And limit it to 2 ounces a day so you don't overindulge in the fat and calories that come along with dark chocolate's healthy natural chemicals. Pick your favorite treat:

- 12 dark chocolate Hershey Kisses
- 7 pieces of Dove dark chocolate miniatures
- 6 tablespoons of cocoa powder made into hot chocolate

For more information on helping your heart with chocolate, see "Sweet way to stave off heart disease" in the *Heart disease* chapter.

Milk does your body good

Following the DASH eating plan can help in your fight against high blood pressure, and part of the reason is the two to three daily servings of dairy products included. Milk benefits your blood pressure in several ways.

Protein. Research shows getting 40 grams (g) daily of either milk or soy proteins can bring down systolic pressure — the first, or higher, number in a blood pressure reading. When people with high-normal or slightly elevated blood pressure added the protein to their diets for just eight weeks, their blood pressure improved — unlike folks who took 40 g of a refined carbohydrate supplement instead.

Calcium. This important mineral helps remove excess sodium from your body through your urine. And that's not all. Filling your glass with milk helps you avoid the extra sugar in sweetened beverages like sodas, sweet tea, and sweetened fruit drinks. Cutting back on processed sugar, along with other healthy-eating changes, brought down high blood pressure in three-quarters of the people in one study. It took just a couple of months to see the benefits.

Pick low-fat or skim milk for the greatest effect on your blood pressure, since saturated fat in other dairy products seems to cancel out the benefits.

HEALTH ALERT!

You probably know to steer clear of grapefruit while you're taking meds for high blood pressure. But that's not the only citrus you need to avoid. Seville oranges — also known as sour or bitter oranges — contain some of the same compounds that can cause dangerous interactions with many prescription drugs. This fruit is typically used to make orange marmalade, so never eat it without talking to your doctor first.

Inflammatory bowel disease

Squelch flare-ups with yogurt

To fight inflammatory bowel disease, your best weapon just might be a spoon. Dip that spoon into some probiotic yogurt, and you'll get a delicious — and potentially helpful — dose of protection.

Inflammatory bowel disease (IBD), which includes both ulcerative colitis and Crohn's disease, can make your life miserable. Ulcerative colitis involves inflammation of the colon and rectum, while Crohn's disease can affect your entire intestinal tract, from mouth to rectum. Symptoms include rectal pain and cramping, bloody diarrhea, stomach pain, nausea, appetite loss, weight loss, and fever.

Thanks to probiotics, yogurt can help. These good bacteria crowd out harmful bacteria in your digestive tract to restore balance. They may also work in other ways to boost your immune system.

Thank protein power. Researchers from Vanderbilt University Medical Center shed some light on how probiotics may work. They isolated a soluble protein from *Lactobacillus rhamnosus GG* (LGG), a probiotic found in yogurt. The protein, called p40, works by activating the epidermal growth factor receptor (EGFR). When activated, EGFR protects colon cells from apoptosis, or cell death, and from chronic inflammation that can weaken defenses against bad bacteria in the bloodstream. In tests performed on mice, p40 prevented and treated colitis.

Enjoy encouraging evidence. An earlier study found that combining a commercial product called VSL#3, a blend of several strains of probiotics, with balsalazide, a drug commonly used to treat ulcerative colitis, worked better than higher doses of the drug by itself. By the end of the yearlong study, 24 out of the 30 people who took the combination were in remission.

> Sprinkle your yogurt with blueberries for an extra boost. Swedish researchers found that blueberry fiber protects against intestinal inflammation — and blueberries work even better when paired with probiotics.

Other studies have found that probiotics may help treat diarrhea caused by Crohn's disease and prevent pouchitis, a common complication of a surgical procedure to remove the colon in people with severe ulcerative colitis. However, more research is needed before probiotics become a standard treatment for IBD.

Seek out super snacks. In the meantime, eat more yogurt to reap the benefits of probiotics. Make sure your yogurt contains live active cultures. Look for yogurts that provide at least 10 billion colony forming units (CFU) per serving.

You can also find probiotic supplements, but because they are not regulated by the FDA, you can't be sure you're getting what the label claims — plus, they don't taste as good as smooth, creamy yogurt.

Get tasty relief from grapes

Feel imprisoned by inflammatory bowel disease? Make a "grape" escape. Grapes and grape juice contain a powerful compound called resveratrol, an antioxidant that fights inflammation and boosts your immune system. Spanish researchers have found that resveratrol helps treat ulcerative colitis in mice.

Experience fewer symptoms. In the study, mice were fed either a standard diet or a diet supplemented with resveratrol. Then they were given a drug to bring on acute colitis, which advanced to chronic intestinal inflammation. The mice on the resveratrol diet showed fewer symptoms, including loss of body weight, diarrhea, and rectal bleeding. All of them also survived the treatment, while 40 percent of the mice on the standard diet did not.

Three weeks after the mice were taken off the drug, those in the resveratrol group had lower levels of pro-inflammatory cytokines and higher levels of an anti-inflammatory cytokine. Other telltale signs of inflammation also appeared lower in the resveratrol group. Of course, what works for mice may not work for humans — but these results are promising.

HEALTH ALERT!

Carnivores beware! A high intake of meat may mean a higher risk of developing inflammatory bowel disease. That's what a large French study discovered.

Researchers tracked the eating habits of 67,581 French women ages 40 to 65 for an average of more than 10 years. Women who ate the most protein — especially animal protein — were three times more likely to develop IBD than those who ate the least. Results were similar for both Crohn's disease and ulcerative colitis.

But not all animal protein was bad. Eating lots of meat and fish seemed to boost the risk of IBD, but large amounts of eggs and dairy products did not. You don't have to cut out meat entirely, but it can't hurt to cut back. Minimizing your meat intake may minimize your IBD risk.

Take advantage of food sources. To get the equivalent amount of resveratrol as the mice in the study, a 150-pound person would need about 30 milligrams (mg) a day. That's more than you'd get through a reasonable diet. For example, a cup of grapes would give you at most 1.25 mg of resveratrol, while a 5-ounce glass of grape juice may provide as much as 1.3 mg.

But it can't hurt to boost your intake of resveratrol-rich foods. Besides grapes and grape juice, you can find resveratrol in red wine, peanuts, and some berries, including blueberries and cranberries. The amount of resveratrol in foods and beverages can vary greatly, so it's hard to tell exactly how much you'll get.

You can also find resveratrol in supplement form, but you should check with your doctor before taking any supplements. Stick with grapes and other food sources of resveratrol for now. It could be a tasty way to combat ulcerative colitis.

Apples take aim against inflammation

Here's an easy way to grapple with inflammatory bowel disease. Bite into an apple. Just make sure to eat the peel. Apple peels contain polyphenols, antioxidants with anti-inflammatory powers. And a study out of Montana State University determined that apple polyphenols helped prevent colitis in mice.

Mice received either apple polyphenols or a placebo after researchers used chemicals to bring on colitis. Those who got the apple polyphenols warded off the disease, avoiding symptoms such as weight loss and inflammation of the colon. Apple polyphenols appear to fight inflammation by suppressing T-cell activation. In fact, T cells seem to be the key to polyphenols' success. In mice lacking these cells, the apple polyphenols did not help.

This study could lead to new treatments for inflammatory bowel disease. But in the meantime, why not enjoy an occasional apple?

This healthy and delicious fruit makes a perfect snack. And when it comes to IBD, an apple may help you get to the "core" of the problem.

Brew up this soothing remedy for IBD

Thousands of years ago, tea was thought to be one of the most potent medicines. Today, modern researchers are once again exploring tea's healing properties. They've found evidence to suggest that the polyphenols in green tea can help thwart inflammatory bowel disease (IBD).

A paper published in the journal *Nutrients* suggests green tea compounds can fight inflammation and relieve symptoms in IBD sufferers. And other research found that drinking a cup of tea every day was linked with a lower risk of developing IBD.

Experts think the most powerful polyphenol in tea is epigallocatechin gallate (EGCG). This natural chemical breaks down as tea gets older, so aged teas — like black or oolong — have less of it. But before you bring out the kettle, you should know that cold steeping tea may be even healthier. That's because brewing in boiling water will destroy some of tea's natural antioxidants.

Oil change wards off colitis

Worried about developing ulcerative colitis? Fat chance — as long as you choose the right kind of fat. Studies suggest that certain fatty acids may reduce your risk, while others could increase it.

Opt for oleic acid. This heart-healthy monounsaturated fatty acid, found in olive oil, blocks the formation of compounds that aggravate inflammation in your colon. In a British study of more than 25,000 people, those whose diets contained the most oleic acid had an 89 percent lower risk of developing ulcerative colitis during the nearly four years of follow-up.

Researchers estimated that 46 percent of ulcerative colitis cases could be prevented if people consumed more oleic acid. Just 2 to 3 tablespoons of olive oil a day should do the trick.

Limit linoleic acid. On the other hand, some fatty acids aren't so good. In an earlier study, British researchers found that a high intake of linoleic acid, an omega-6 fatty acid found in vegetable oils, may boost your risk of developing ulcerative colitis.

In the study, which tracked the eating habits of more than 200,000 people for an average of four years, those whose diets contained the most linoleic acid were more than twice as likely to develop ulcerative colitis as those who ate the least. Unlike oleic acid, linoleic acid produces pro-inflammatory substances that can wreak havoc in your colon.

Make the switch. Swap your vegetable oil for olive oil, and you may get a double dose of protection. This simple oil change could be an easy way to lower your risk of developing ulcerative colitis.

Besides olive oil, other good sources of oleic acid include grapeseed oil, peanut oil, and avocados. You can mash some avocados to make homemade guacamole or add fresh avocado slices to sandwiches or salads.

Insomnia

Chase away insomnia with cherries

Trouble sleeping? Try this fruit. Scientists say you could get all the sleep-inducing melatonin you need in a handful of tart cherries.

That's important because melatonin plays a key role in regulating your sleep-wake cycle. This hormone is produced by your brain's pineal gland, but it's also found in some foods and is available as a dietary supplement. Studies have shown that melatonin supplements may help treat insomnia, jet lag, and other sleep disturbances.

Tart cherries provide a natural — and tasty — way to boost your melatonin levels. Before turning to supplements, give this fruit a try. These tart treats may lead to sweet dreams.

Juicy developments. Two studies explored the effects of tart cherry juice on sleep — and the results look promising.

A small University of Rochester study determined that tart cherry juice can modestly improve sleep in older people with insomnia. In the study, 15 people with an average age of more than 71 years drank two 8-ounce glasses of tart cherry juice or a placebo beverage each day, once in the morning between 8 a.m. and 10 a.m. and once at night, one to two hours before bedtime. The cherry juice provided the equivalent of about 100 tart cherries a day.

However, the study didn't explore how the cherry juice worked. Researchers noted that either melatonin or the anti-inflammatory properties of cherries could get the credit.

In a British study, 20 volunteers drank either tart cherry juice concentrate or a placebo for seven days. Those in the cherry juice group had significantly elevated levels of melatonin by the study's end. They also slept longer and better.

Cherry choices. Besides drinking tart cherry juice, you can also find frozen or dried tart cherries in your supermarket year-round. It's easy to fit more of them into your diet. Just sprinkle some of the dried fruit into your yogurt, oatmeal, or salads.

Other foods that contain melatonin include oats, sweet corn, rice, ginger, tomatoes, bananas, and barley. Experiment to see which ones work best for you.

HEALTH ALERT!

Insomnia doesn't just leave you tired the next day. Poor sleep may raise your blood pressure and lead to heart disease or stroke. It may even speed up mental decline. Lack of sleep has also been linked to colon cancer. As the severity of your sleep problems increase, so does your risk of developing fibromyalgia.

Sleeping less may lead to eating more, boosting your risk of obesity and related health problems. When you don't get enough sleep, you may find it harder to resist tempting foods or to lose weight.

It's not just your health or your waistline that's at stake — it's your money, too. Lack of sleep may spur you to make riskier financial decisions.

Combo keeps sleep-wake cycle in balance

"Night and Day," Cole Porter's popular contribution to the Great American Songbook, also serves as a good reminder of the sleep-wake cycle. In order to sleep well at night, you need to be awake and expend energy during the day. After expending energy all day, you should be tired at night so you sleep well and feel refreshed the next day.

Making the right food choices can help this cycle continue. Discover three foods that will keep your body awake — and two foods that will help you sleep.

Perk up with protein. Keep your body awake during the day by choosing high-protein foods. Protein may promote wakefulness by boosting the activity of catecholamines, brain messengers like adrenaline involved in the body's "fight-or-flight" response. Good choices include meat, eggs, and low-fat dairy products.

Calm down with carbs. To wind down at night, switch to foods rich in carbohydrates. An Australian study found that starchy carbohydrates eaten four hours before bedtime helped people fall asleep faster. That's because these carbohydrates may boost levels of tryptophan and serotonin, two brain chemicals involved in sleep. The study used jasmine rice, but pasta should also do the trick.

You can also try other types of carbohydrates that rank high on the Glycemic Index, which measures how quickly foods raise your blood sugar. Good options include mashed potatoes, bagels, saltine or graham crackers, pretzels, and rice cakes.

Conquer sleep woes with chamomile

Stop spending big bucks for drugs that help you sleep. Your spice rack is packed with herbal healing power. Reach for chamomile to help you get a good night's rest.

This traditional sleep remedy, usually taken in the form of tea, helps you relax. Chamomile contains a natural plant compound called apigenin, which has a mild sedative effect. It works by binding to the same receptors as benzodiazepines, drugs that were once commonly used to treat insomnia and anxiety.

One study of heart surgery patients accidentally discovered that chamomile tea may help promote sleep, as 10 out of 12 people fell asleep shortly after drinking it. Although more research is needed to confirm this finding, feel free to give chamomile a try.

A soothing cup of chamomile tea may put you on the road to dreamland. To make your own tea, steep 1 heaping teaspoon of dried chamomile flowers in hot water for 10 minutes. You can drink up to 3 cups a day.

Just be careful. If you are allergic to ragweed, steer clear of chamomile, which comes from the same family.

Discover a hidden cause of insomnia

You may blame a lumpy mattress or your husband's snoring if you spend all night tossing and turning. But believe it or not, the blame may lie with your bedclothes. Wearing tight-fitting underwear or a bra to bed could cause discomfort that keeps you up all night. These garments may even hinder circulation, put pressure on your chest, and make it difficult to breathe. Instead, opt for loose-fitting pajamas. Stay comfortable by sleeping in fabrics like cotton, silk, and bamboo.

Discover the power of kiwifruit

Tired of lying in bed waiting for sleep to come? Eat some kiwifruit. This unusual fruit may also serve as an unusual sleep aid.

A Taiwanese study found that eating kiwifruit can help people with sleep disorders. In the study, 24 people ages 20 to 55 ate two kiwis 60 minutes before bedtime each night for four weeks. They fell asleep faster, slept longer, and slept better after eating this tasty treat.

Named for the hairy, flightless national bird of New Zealand, kiwifruit contains plenty of compounds that may help you sleep, including antioxidants, serotonin, and folate.

- Antioxidants. Sleep disorders and stress can boost the concentration of harmful free radicals in your body. Loaded with antioxidants like vitamin C, kiwis may counteract these damaging substances. Flavonoids, anthocyanins, and carotenoids may also contribute to the fruit's antioxidant powers.
- Serotonin. Low levels of the neurotransmitter serotonin may cause insomnia. Luckily, kiwis packs plenty of serotonin into a tiny package.
- Folate. A deficiency of this key B vitamin may also trigger insomnia. Kiwifruit not only provides plenty of folate, but because you eat it raw, you don't lose any during cooking or processing.

This promising study suggests that kiwifruit can be a tasty way to improve the quality of your sleep. Look for kiwis in the produce section of your supermarket.

About the size and shape of a large hen's egg, kiwifruit has a hairy, dull-brown skin. Inside, it sports emerald green flesh, with rows of black, edible seeds. These seeds give kiwifruit a texture similar to a strawberry. Kiwis taste like a blend of strawberry, pineapple, and sweet melon. You can eat the fuzzy skin, but you probably don't want to. Before eating kiwifruit, cut off the tips and peel the skin with a vegetable peeler.

Kiwifruit tastes great by itself, but it can also spruce up several other foods. Slices of kiwifruit brighten up your fruit salads, while kiwi wedges can garnish any meal. Serve a spicy kiwi salsa over meat, or add kiwifruit to fish, poultry, or meat dishes. Kiwifruit also goes well with avocado, radicchio, and endive. For a refreshing drink, combine fresh kiwi puree, orange juice, and sparkling water. You can also use kiwifruit in pies, puddings, and breads. For a tasty dessert, try topping your ice cream with kiwi sauce or slices.

Did you know?

A squirt of mustard can wallop your nighttime leg cramps. That's right — the spicy spread eases those painful muscle contractions that can make it difficult to fall back to sleep.

Historians believe the Romans were the first to mix mustard seeds and wine or vinegar to make a paste. Then French monks got in on the act, combining ground mustard seeds with unfermented wine and naming it "mustard," from the Latin for "burning wine."

Delicious, yes. But can it help relieve leg cramps, too? You bet, according to experts. Prepared mustard contains vinegar and sodium, the same muscle-soothing ingredients found in sports drinks and the trendy cramp reliever, pickle juice. And bright yellow turmeric — added to give mustard its appealing color — is bursting with anti-inflammatory properties that might be just what the doctor ordered for your late-night muscle cramps. A couple of teaspoons is all you need to stop a charley horse in its tracks.

Irritable bowel syndrome

Minty method to soothe symptoms

Irritable bowel syndrome (IBS) sure can make you irritable. But you don't have to suffer with gas, cramping, stomach pain, bloating, constipation, diarrhea, and other symptoms. Peppermint will give you relief. This old, common folk remedy for tummy troubles has plenty of science on its side. Several studies suggest that peppermint oil relieves symptoms of IBS.

Examine the evidence. One review of 38 IBS studies — including four dealing with peppermint oil — determined that peppermint was an effective treatment, helping 74 percent of study participants. That compares favorably with other remedies, such as antispasmodics and fiber.

A more recent review focused on two strong studies. In one, peppermint oil capsules significantly improved IBS symptoms after four weeks of treatment when compared with a placebo. Two capsules containing 225 milligrams (mg) of peppermint oil, taken twice daily, helped relieve constipation, bloating, diarrhea, stomach pain, gas, and pain while using the toilet.

In the other study, which lasted eight weeks, people who took a capsule containing 187 mg of peppermint oil three times a day saw significant improvements in stomach pain and overall quality of life compared to those taking a placebo.

Curb contractions. Experts believe peppermint oil works by reducing spasms in the smooth muscles of your digestive tract. It may do this by blocking the flow of calcium into these muscle cells. As a result, you experience less stomach pain, cramping, and bloating. Peppermint oil may also work by activating a specific "anti-pain" channel in the large intestine.

Pick up some peppermint. Look for enteric-coated peppermint oil capsules at your local big-box store or drugstore. It's best to take them before meals to ease intestinal distress. Just make sure to consult your doctor before taking any supplements. You can also try sipping peppermint tea or sucking on a peppermint candy for a tasty dose of relief.

Take action against IBS

Boosting your physical activity can help relieve symptoms of irritable bowel syndrome (IBS). It also helps prevent IBS symptoms from getting worse.

That's what Swedish researchers discovered. Half of the people in their study were encouraged to exercise more, while the others were told to maintain their current lifestyles. At the start of the study, and again three months later, both groups rated their symptoms using the IBS Severity Scoring System.

Those in the exercise group lowered their scores by 51 points, compared to 5 points for the control group. While 23 percent of the control group reported more severe symptoms, only 8 percent of the exercise group reported worsening symptoms.

Get moving, and you'll help get your IBS symptoms under control. Aim for 20 to 30 minutes of low- to moderate-intensity exercise three to five times per week.

Protect yourself with probiotics

Irritable bowel syndrome (IBS) comes with plenty of cons. Counteract them with some pros — probiotics. These "good bacteria" can restore order to your digestive tract and boost your natural defenses.

Fight IBS symptoms such as bloating, constipation, and diarrhea, and prevent sinus infections, urinary tract infections, and eczema — all with one supplement. Discover how probiotics can help and how you can make them part of your diet.

Benefit your bowels. Several studies suggest that probiotics help relieve IBS symptoms. Various strains of *Lactobacillus* and *Bifidobacterium* seem to have the most beneficial effects. These probiotics help reduce bloating, abdominal pain, and gas in people with IBS. They may also help promote regularity, increasing the number of bowel movements for constipated women and decreasing them for those with diarrhea.

Probiotics likely work by restoring the proper balance of bacteria in your digestive tract. Antibiotics can kill good as well as bad bacteria, which explains why taking antibiotics may result in diarrhea. Luckily, probiotics can help reduce the risk of antibiotic-associated diarrhea. Probiotics, along with drinking extra water, also help shorten a bout of acute diarrhea.

Conquer other conditions. Probiotics can protect more than your gut. Evidence suggests that they can also help ward off the following conditions.

- Sinus infections. Swiss researchers found that drinking a probiotic fermented milk drink daily for three weeks helped lower the number of potentially pathogenic bacteria (PPBs) in the nose. These harmful bacteria can cause sinus infections and pneumonia, among other problems. Other studies have found that probiotics can help shorten the length and severity of the common cold and the length of winter infections in older people.

- Urinary tract infections. Studies suggest that probiotics, specifically *lactobacilli*, can help prevent recurrent urinary tract infections in women. They likely work by keeping the pH of the vagina low and preventing the growth of harmful bacteria.
- Eczema. Also known as atopic dermatitis, eczema is a chronic skin condition featuring itching, redness, swelling, dryness, and scaling. Probiotics may play a role in preventing eczema in young children, according to a few studies.

Seek out sources. You can find probiotics in several forms. Probiotic supplements come in capsules, powders, tablets, and liquid form. As always, make sure to consult your doctor before taking any supplements.

You can also find probiotics in certain foods, mostly yogurt and milk. Two of the more common probiotic products include Activia, a probiotic yogurt, and DanActive, a fermented dairy drink. Probiotics may also pop up in granola bars, miso, cereals, and juices. Check labels to make sure you're getting live bacteria and a high count of "colony forming units," or CFU. Aim for at least 10 billion CFU per serving.

Say cheese. Did you know that choosing the right kind of cheese can boost your immune system, protecting you from infections, inflammation, even cancer? A Finnish study discovered that probiotic cheese can help fight age-related changes to your immune system that leave you more vulnerable to these dangers.

Researchers gave older people living in the same nursing home a slice of Gouda cheese with breakfast each day for 10 weeks. One group switched to probiotic cheese during a four-week span, while the other group continued to eat Gouda. Blood tests determined that those who ate the probiotic cheese had improved immune response.

However you get your probiotics — from supplements, yogurt, milk, or cheese — you'll fight IBS symptoms and other conditions like a pro.

Dynamic duo guards your health

Probiotic yogurts and fermented dairy drinks do more than fight irritable bowel syndrome. These foods can help fight diabetes, high blood pressure, gout, and infections. So be sure to get some next time you're at the supermarket.

One study found that higher blood levels of a compound called trans-palmitoleic acid, found in whole-fat dairy products, may substantially lower your risk of developing type 2 diabetes. Another found that milk protein lowers systolic blood pressure, the top number in a blood pressure reading. Eating dairy has also been shown to decrease the risk of developing gout. Aim for one to two servings of dairy a day.

Sing away your stress

Irritable bowel syndrome (IBS) can leave you feeling out of tune with your body. Here's a fun way to get back in harmony — sing.

Swedish researchers examined the effects of choir singing, a popular pastime in Nordic countries, on people with IBS. In one study, researchers took the study participants' saliva samples to measure stress levels.

After six months, samples from the choir group had higher concentrations of testosterone, a sign that their bodies were recovering from stress. Since stress can trigger or worsen IBS symptoms, that's a good sign. Although the effect disappeared after one year, the weekly choir sessions helped in the short term.

In a previous study, researchers found that singing lessons helped promote feelings of relaxation, energy, and joy. Singing also boosts levels of the feel-good hormone oxytocin, which may fight pain. If you have IBS, that should be music to your ears.

Meanwhile, probiotics may help you ward off infections — including colds, sinusitis, and urinary tract problems — as well as shorten the time you spend dealing with diarrhea. So it's easy to see that you get the best of both worlds by eating and drinking probiotic yogurts and fermented dairy drinks.

Incredible antidote for indigestion

Upset stomach? Bypass your medicine cabinet and reach for the spice rack. You'll find a surprising but reliable remedy — cinnamon.

HEALTH ALERT!

Bothersome bowels? You can find foods that soothe — and foods that irritate. Watch out for foods that can make IBS symptoms worse. For some people, that includes:

- wheat, dairy products, eggs, coffee, yeast, potatoes, or citrus fruits.
- fructose-filled soft drinks, cereals, and packaged baked goods.
- artificial sweeteners in sugar-free or reduced-sugar foods.

One eating plan, called the low-FODMAP (fermentable oligosaccharides, disaccharides, monosaccharides, and polyols) diet, is worth noting. Developed in Australia, this diet eliminates foods high in sugars that can be difficult to digest and then gradually reintroduces them to see what your body can tolerate.

One study found that a low-FODMAP diet greatly improved symptoms like bloating, abdominal pain, and gas. This diet can be tricky to follow, though, because so many foods contain FODMAP sugars. For best results, you may want to work with a dietitian.

You know cinnamon adds an aromatic punch to pies, cobblers, and other treats. But did you know that this spice can also relieve indigestion?

That's what practitioners of herbal medicine have known for years. Ayurvedic and traditional Chinese medicine make use of cinnamon to treat digestive disorders, including indigestion, gas, and diarrhea. Ancient Greeks and Romans also used this spice for better digestion.

Even today, it's recommended by herbalists to soothe indigestion, bloating, and gas. Although scientists can't tell you how it works, it might have to do with the way cinnamon warms up your stomach and helps stimulate digestion.

While there have been few human studies to support the medicinal use of cinnamon, it can't hurt to add a few dashes of this delightful spice to your meals. Try sprinkling ground cinnamon on cooked carrots, winter squash, sweet potatoes, or your morning oatmeal. Or swizzle cinnamon sticks in hot cider, coffee drinks, or juices.

Perking up your foods and beverages with a little extra cinnamon could mean a little less indigestion for you.

Focus on the right fiber

Boosting your fiber intake may help ward off digestive disorders like irritable bowel syndrome. But if you already have IBS, choose your fiber wisely.

Get psyched for psyllium. This soluble fiber, also known as ispaghula husk, seems to provide the most relief for people with IBS.

Dutch researchers compared the effects of psyllium, bran, and a placebo (rice flour) on IBS symptoms. People in the 12-week study took 10 grams of their assigned fiber supplement each day, divided into two doses mixed with food.

Psyllium performed best, helping a greater percentage of people and reducing symptom severity by 90 points compared with 58 for bran and 49 for the placebo. An earlier review of six studies also deemed psyllium an effective treatment for IBS.

Ban bran. Bran did not fare nearly as well. In fact, bran may actually worsen symptoms. In the Dutch study, many people dropped out of the bran group for this reason. And a review of five studies found that bran worked no better than a placebo or a low-fiber diet.

Shop for soluble fiber. As a soluble fiber, psyllium likely works by slowing the rate at which your stomach empties. You may be familiar with a brand of psyllium called Metamucil. You can buy this and other brands at big-box stores or online. Mix it with water or add it to foods like yogurt. It's also available in capsule form.

Other good sources of soluble fiber include apples, citrus fruits, peas, beans, carrots, flaxseed, oats, and barley. An animal study suggests that pectin, a form of soluble fiber found in apples, improves gut health.

Did you know?

Looking for an exciting new source of fiber? Go green. Freekeh, a Middle Eastern grain, refers to wheat harvested when the grain is still young, or green.

Freekeh, which boasts four times more fiber than brown rice, helps prevent constipation and manage symptoms of irritable bowel syndrome. It also encourages the growth of good bacteria in your digestive tract.

Look for freekeh in your local health food store. Enjoy it as a hot cereal, a side dish like rice or pasta, or a tasty addition to soups and salads.

Kidney stones

Make a DASH for healthy kidneys

You can keep your kidneys functioning and avoid painful kidney stones by eating the right foods. Turns out that following the DASH diet — Dietary Approaches to Stop Hypertension — also cuts down on your risk of developing kidney stones.

Banish the pain. A kidney stone occurs when minerals in your urine form into crystals. Most of the time stones pass harmlessly into the bladder and out of your body, often without pain. But larger stones can cause serious pain as they pass, and you may also notice blood in your urine, nausea, vomiting, fever, and chills. If you've had one kidney stone, you have a 50 percent chance of suffering from another one within a decade.

DASH to protection. To see how the DASH diet might help prevent kidney stones, researchers looked at information from more than 240,000 men and women who participated in either the Health Professionals Follow-up Study or the Nurses' Health Studies I and II. Some folks had suffered from kidney stones, while others had not.

People who more strictly followed the DASH diet for up to 18 years were much less likely to have suffered from kidney stones. The most strict DASH followers reported eating more calcium, potassium, magnesium, oxalate, and vitamin C, while they ate less sodium. Interestingly, the higher levels of oxalate didn't seem to cause more stones, as might be expected.

Other research looked at people following the DASH diet and found these kidney benefits:

- higher levels of calcium and citrate in urine
- greater volumes of urine passed
- more potassium, magnesium, and phosphate in urine
- higher urine pH

These positive results show how the DASH diet may help protect you from kidney stones.

Follow the plan. The DASH diet was designed to help bring down blood pressure but it's a healthy eating plan whether you have blood pressure problems or not. If you have a tendency toward kidney stones, it may be worth trying.

Focus on eating lots of whole grains, fruits, vegetables, nuts, legumes, and low-fat dairy. People following the DASH eating plan also try to avoid too much sodium, sweetened beverages, and red and processed meats.

Vegetables are an important part of the DASH diet, but some are naturally high in oxalates. Limit these high-oxalate favorites if you tend to form calcium oxalate kidney stones, and you may steer clear of the problem.

- spinach
- beet greens
- okra
- leeks
- collard greens
- parsley
- potatoes

You're safer eating kale or turnip greens, which contain lower levels of oxalates.

Did you know?

Most kidney stones contain calcium. So you may have heard you shouldn't take calcium supplements if you tend to develop kidney stones. Research varies on whether supplemental calcium can contribute to painful stones.

But some evidence shows getting lots of calcium from the foods you eat may actually lower your risk of kidney stones. So eat plenty of high-calcium foods like low-fat milk, yogurt, and cheese, and ask your doctor whether a calcium supplement is a good idea for you.

Surprising drinks that dissolve kidney stones

People who tend to form kidney stones need to drink lots of fluids — as much as 12 cups a day — to dissolve minerals that can end up in urine. Drinking water is great, but that can get boring. Besides, certain beverages actually beat water when it comes to preventing kidney stones.

Enjoy a citrus thirst quencher. Some people prone to stones have too little citrate in their urine. This condition allows calcium to bind to free oxalate or phosphate to form a stone. Sometimes doctors prescribe citrate supplements, but drinking lemonade is another way to raise your citrate levels. Be sure to drink lemonade made with natural lemon juice for the best results.

Here's another reason to lose those extra pounds. Obese people — body mass index (BMI) of 30 or higher — have a much higher risk of developing kidney stones compared to thinner folks.

Don't forget your morning OJ. Good old orange juice also raises the citrate levels in urine. Researchers found that women who drank up to about a quart of orange juice daily had less urine acidity and more citric acid excretion. These changes greatly lower your risk of forming calcium oxalate stones.

Other research found that, although grapefruit juice has lots of citrate, it may not do much to lower your risk of kidney stones. In fact, drinking grapefruit juice may do more harm than good. One study found drinking 8 ounces of grapefruit juice per day could raise your risk of a stone by 44 percent.

Mix coffee just right. Add a little milk to your coffee and tea to neutralize the oxalates. Milk binds to free oxalates, so you won't need to worry about these stone-forming compounds.

Switch it up with diet soda. In an effort to find drinks that people really enjoy, researchers checked citrate levels in various sodas. Certain diet citrus sodas, including Diet 7Up, Sprite Zero, and Diet Mountain Dew, actually contained more citrate than even lemonade. But dark-colored sodas like Coke Zero and Diet Pepsi had lower citrate levels. So you'll want to stick to light-colored diet sodas for the best protection.

Treat your kidney stones with bananas

You can thank your kidneys for creating urine from the waste and excess water in your blood. But sometimes things go wrong, and minerals and salts start to build up. Next thing you know, you have kidney stones.

Stones can also form when acid levels in urine grow too high. That's why some experts believe high levels of potassium, which is an alkaline that neutralizes acids, could lower your risk of developing kidney stones. Lucky for you, a single banana has 375 milligrams of potassium. That's more than 10% of the amount you should get each day. No drugs needed!

Liver disease

Keep your body safe from toxic waste

Imitation pancake syrup won't protect your body from bacteria and toxins, but pure maple syrup might. That may sound strange, but some research suggests that maple syrup may have more to offer than just sugar.

A University of Tokyo study compared animals on a diet of 20 percent pure maple syrup to animals getting a mix of sugars similar to it. The maple syrup group scored better on liver function tests. What's more, the genes that encouraged the production of toxic ammonia — produced by your body when proteins are digested — were less active. That means less ammonia and less toxic waste for your liver to process.

Other studies have found that pure maple syrup contains plenty of nutrients, including zinc, calcium, antioxidants, and more than 50 phytonutrients. But this doesn't mean you should eat it at every meal. Just 1 tablespoon equals half the 100-calorie a day limit of added sugar — 150 for men — recommended by the American Heart Association.

On the other hand, if you enjoy pancakes occasionally, don't settle for cheap substitutes with maple flavoring or traces of maple syrup mixed in. Instead, try a little bit of pure maple syrup, so you get valuable nutrients along with the sweet taste.

While pure maple syrup might protect your liver from too much toxic ammonia, your liver also protects you from other toxins and dangerous bacteria. As blood flow enters your liver from the

Did you know?

Basil fresh from your garden is wonderful, but holy basil *(Ocimum sanctum)* may be even better. For centuries, folks claimed holy basil could keep you young. Modern research from India suggests that claim may not be just another empty promise.

Research results presented by scientists at the British Pharmaceutical Conference suggest holy basil extract is an antioxidant that helps seek out and destroy free radicals. It even helps preserve crucial organs like your heart, liver, and brain from the free radical damage that contributes to disease and aging.

Today holy basil is widely used to make herbal or medicinal tea in many parts of Asia, but its future role in health may be much more exciting — so stay tuned.

rest of your digestive tract, your liver sends out its defenders, the Kupffer cells. These cells nab bacteria and toxins from your bloodstream, inactivate them, and release them for elimination from your body.

Here's how you can keep your liver running smoothly to make sure the Kupffer cells keep filtering out bacteria and toxins.

- Limit alcohol.
- Lose weight gradually if you are overweight. This helps fight fatty liver disease. Look for high-flavor, low-calorie foods to help.
- Limit cholesterol and saturated fats, particularly from fast foods, meat, and high-fat dairy foods. Substitute whole grains and produce.

- Get active if you are sedentary, but seek your doctor's permission first.
- Find out if any over-the-counter and prescription drugs you take may cause liver damage. Read the labels and product inserts, then talk to your doctor or pharmacist and follow his advice.

A pinch of protection from a zesty spice

You may be absorbing cancer-causing substances without even knowing it. Eating processed meat, using certain cosmetics, or being around secondhand smoke can expose you to a cancer-causing substance called diethylnitrosamine (DEN). DEN may raise your risk of liver cancer, especially if you already have fatty liver disease, chronic hepatitis, or drink alcohol heavily.

Fortunately, research suggests making simple changes in what you eat and how you live could help you fight cancer-causing compounds, detoxify your liver, and prevent cancer. Even little things like the spices you use may make a difference.

Research suggests that one spice, saffron, may help reduce your danger of liver cancer. Asian researchers found that animals that developed liver cancer from DEN fared better if they were given saffron every day. Here is what saffron did to protect them:

- helped prevent cancer cells from multiplying
- contributed to apoptosis, a defense mechanism that makes cancer cells self-destruct
- helped protect against cancer by blocking inflammation
- inhibited the development of cells tainted with compounds that help cancer cells develop and grow

Not surprisingly, animals given saffron developed fewer liver cancer nodules. Even better, animals that were given saffron before liver cancer developed had lower levels of the proteins that indicate liver damage.

More research is needed to find out whether saffron can work in humans. But that's not all researchers want to know. The animals in the study were given large amounts of saffron. Future studies may reveal how much saffron is needed to keep your liver healthy.

Meanwhile, start cooking with saffron. Although this spice is famous for being very expensive, you don't need much. A tiny amount goes a long way. Too much saffron makes food taste bitter.

For an interesting side dish, try adding 1/2 teaspoon of saffron to the water you use to cook 2 cups of rice. The resulting bright flavor may delight you. Saffron is also delicious in vegetable sautés, soups, curries, stews, paellas, and tomato sauces. This spice is very popular in Europe, India, southwestern Asia, and Turkey.

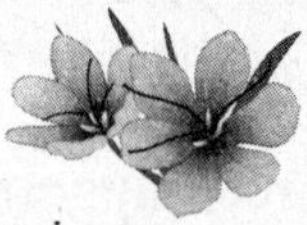

Choose wisely when buying saffron. Threads of saffron, the stigma of a certain crocus flower, are more expensive. Powdered saffron is often a mix of saffron and cheaper ingredients. If you choose the pricier saffron threads, use this trick to reap the most value from them.

Soak the threads for 15 minutes in water, broth, or wine that's hot — but not boiling, or for several hours in cool liquid. If possible, choose a liquid that is an ingredient in your recipe. Add both the liquid and threads to your dish. This draws more flavor from the threads, and it helps distribute saffron's color evenly throughout your dish.

Lung cancer

Take a bite out of lung cancer

Bite into a crunchy, delicious apple, and you just might lower your risk of lung cancer and other serious lung problems. Find out how the proverbial "apple a day" can keep your lungs functioning like they're designed to — and more.

Chances are you associate lung cancer with cigarette smoking. While smoking is still the biggest risk factor for lung cancer, lung cancer among nonsmokers is on the rise. In fact, nonsmokers and people who have smoked fewer than 100 cigarettes in their lifetime account for about 10 to 20 percent of lung cancer cases in the United States. Nonsmoking women are also more likely to get lung cancer than men who don't smoke.

Boost your defenses. If you smoke, quitting will help lower your risk. Avoiding exposure to secondhand smoke, radon gas, asbestos, and harmful pollutants also helps. But you can also boost your defense with a healthy diet. Start by eating more apples.

A University of Hawaii study found that eating apples and onions — both good food sources of the flavonoid quercetin — reduced the risk of developing lung cancer. Those who ate the most apples reduced their risk by 40 percent compared to those who ate the least. Quercetin has been shown to thwart cancerous tumors in rats and mice. In lab tests, it also blocked the activation of certain carcinogens, or cancer-causing substances.

Calm COPD symptoms. Other studies have found that apples can help with chronic obstructive pulmonary disease (COPD), which includes emphysema and chronic bronchitis. Symptoms include chronic cough, phlegm, and breathlessness.

In a study of people in Singapore, apples reduced these chronic respiratory symptoms. The dietary fiber in apples may lower blood sugar concentrations, which reduces inflammation and boosts antioxidant activity. Flavonoids in apples, including quercetin and catechin, may also protect your lungs because of their antioxidant and anti-inflammatory powers.

Dutch researchers also determined that apples had a beneficial effect on lung function and COPD symptoms. Because a high catechin intake also seemed to help, the catechins in apples could get the credit. However, tea — despite being the richest source of catechins — had no such effect. That means apples could owe their lung-boosting ability to something else.

Whether it's because of the fiber or the flavonoids, apples seem to protect your lungs. But that's not the only reason to eat more of them. These fruits can also reduce your risk of heart attack and stroke, lower your cholesterol, guard against cancer, protect your joints, and keep you regular.

Go nuts to guard your lungs

Here's a nutty way to prevent lung cancer — eat more pistachios. These tiny treats pack lots of gamma-tocopherol, a form of vitamin E that may reduce the risk of lung cancer. Aim for about 2 ounces, or 117 pistachio kernels, each day. Other good sources of gamma-tocopherol include peanuts, pecans, and walnuts.

Migraines

Sniff these spices to nix migraine nausea

Swallowing pills, drinks, or food is the last thing you want to do when dealing with migraine pain and nausea. Fortunately, some people have reported great results from a drug-free remedy that will save you the hassle.

Aromatherapy uses scents from plants to interact with your body and help you feel better. For example, some scents may work with your limbic system to promote relaxation, while others may stimulate production of your body's painkilling endorphins. Some people say peppermint essential oil has helped them ease the nausea of migraines. Some even say the peppermint scent eases their headache pain, too. Try these tactics to see if one works for you.

- Pick up a small vial of peppermint essential oil from a health food or vitamin store. Open the bottle, hold it close enough to smell the cool minty scent, and sniff until you feel better.
- Crush some peppermint leaves, cup them in your hands, and sniff. Keep your face far enough away from the crushed leaves to avoid sniffing them up your nose. Inhale the scent slowly, and then let your breath out slowly. Research suggests this technique of controlled breathing may also help ease the nausea.
- Mix 10 to 15 drops of peppermint essential oil with 6 teaspoons of a neutral carrier oil, such as coconut oil. Add a few drops of this solution to a warm bath. The heat and the peppermint may help settle your stomach.

If peppermint is not right for you, try ginger. Place a few drops of ginger essential oil on a tissue, and sniff until you feel better. Just be careful not to get the essential oil on your hands. If you don't have essential oil, crush fresh ginger into a bowl or shallow glass so you can breathe in its spicy aroma.

Other essential oils recommended for nausea include spearmint, basil, coriander, and fennel. If you choose to try one, remember these safety precautions. Keep essential oils out of your mouth and eyes, and never place undiluted oils directly on your skin. Always dilute essential oils in carrier oils like almond, apricot, grapeseed, or jojoba.

Did you know?

Popping pills every time you get a headache can be a headache in itself. The next time your head throbs, try this "icy–hot" treatment for quick headache relief. Passed down from generation to generation, this folk remedy may sound crazy. But your ancestors would tell you it really works for stress headaches.

While soaking in a steamy bath, hold an ice pack on your head. The combination of hot and cold relieves your headache by drawing blood away from your head and narrowing the blood vessels in your scalp.

If you don't have time for a bath, focus on either a hot or cold technique. Make a hot compress by heating up salt in a dry pan until it's warm, and then pouring the salt into a thin dishtowel and bundling it up. For pain in the front of your head, hold the compress to the back of your head and rub. Wet and freeze old socks in a zip-lock bag to craft a frozen compress.

Osteoarthritis

Curry curbs joint pain

Tired of taking pain relievers for joint pain? Find arthritis relief in your spice rack just by reaching for the turmeric.

This flavorful spice, used in curry, contains a powerful secret weapon called curcumin. Besides giving turmeric its distinctive yellow color, curcumin also provides plenty of benefits.

A Thai study suggests that curcumin can serve as a safe and effective treatment for knee osteoarthritis (OA), working just as well as — and possibly slightly better than — ibuprofen.

In the six-week study of 107 people with knee OA, 52 received 2 grams of curcumin per day and 55 took 800 milligrams of ibuprofen. Participants used a numerical rating scale to assess their pain after walking on level ground or up and down stairs. Researchers also timed them during a 100-meter walk and while going up and down a 10-step flight of stairs.

Results showed that curcumin can relieve pain and improve knee function, as both the pain ratings and time spent on the tasks decreased after six weeks. Curcumin's anti-inflammatory powers likely get the credit, although other studies have shown that curcumin employs multiple mechanisms to protect against inflammation and oxidative damage.

The researchers note that more studies are needed. Specifically, double-blind studies with a larger sample of people and a higher dose of ibuprofen for the comparison group would help make a more convincing case for curcumin as a treatment for OA.

In the meantime, feel free to eat more curry and other dishes that contain turmeric. This herb, with so many health benefits, can actually improve your quality of life.

- Besides its potential to help with osteoarthritis, curcumin has also been shown to reduce inflammation in people with rheumatoid arthritis.
- Thanks to its antioxidant and anti-inflammatory powers, it may also fight chronic conditions like heart disease, type 2 diabetes, cancer, and Alzheimer's disease.
- It also aids digestion and helps with gastrointestinal problems.

Sprinkle some turmeric into your dishes while cooking. You'll give your food an extra kick — and possibly give osteoarthritis pain the boot.

Say goodbye to joint pain

Turmeric isn't the only spice that can help ease joint pain. If you pair it with ginger and cayenne pepper, you'll have three of the top herbal painkillers that really work.

Research suggests that adding about 1/2 teaspoon of ginger to your daily diet can help slash the pain associated with osteoarthritis. As an added bonus, it may help heal your stomach lining, unlike nonsteroidal anti-inflammatory drugs that can damage it.

You may also be able to find relief by turning to cayenne pepper. Experts say capsaicin — the chemical that gives cayenne and other peppers their fiery burn — can help relieve aching joints.

Not a fan of spicy food? No worries. An analysis of 17 studies revealed that topical capsaicin creams are just as effective at battling arthritis pain as over-the-counter medicines.

Sidestep OA with seafood

You may know eating fatty fish like salmon, mackerel, or herring is a simple way to cast off arthritis pain. These foods provide plenty of omega-3 fatty acids, nutrients that work to fight the pain of both osteoarthritis (OA) and rheumatoid arthritis (RA) by reducing inflammation. But a British study suggests that fish may also prevent OA from developing in the first place.

Foil OA before it starts. Researchers from the University of Bristol discovered that a diet rich in omega-3 fatty acids reduced the signs of OA by 50 percent in guinea pigs prone to develop the condition.

The animals received either a high omega-3 diet or a control diet, rich in omega-6 fatty acids. While not bad in and of themselves, omega-6 fatty acids can cause inflammation if you get too much of them. You'll find these fats in corn and soybean oils, margarine, and deep-fried or processed foods — in short, foods that make up a typical Western diet. The high omega-3 diet in the study featured a 1.5:1 ratio of omega 6 to omega 3, while the control diet had a 22:1 ratio.

The omega-3 diet led to beneficial effects on cartilage and bone function. Researchers note that omega-3s may delay or prevent the onset of osteoarthritis. Not only that, these fatty acids may slow its progression. Of course, more studies are needed to confirm these promising results.

The key is to strike a better balance between omega-6 and omega-3 fatty acids. Adjusting your diet could reduce your risk for OA and other inflammatory diseases.

Protect your heart, too. As a bonus, omega-3 fatty acids also help your heart. Studies have shown that they lower blood pressure, bad LDL cholesterol, and triglycerides; slow the buildup of plaque in your arteries; and reduce your risk of arrythmia, or abnormal heartbeat. In fact, the American Heart Association recommends getting two servings of fish per week.

Fatty fish represents the best food source of omega-3 fatty acids, but you can also take fish oil supplements or find other ways to boost your omega-3 intake.

Here are some good sources of omega-3 fatty acids — foods that can help bring down your blood pressure, control your cholesterol, relieve arthritic joints, and perhaps prevent osteoarthritis.

- salmon
- tuna
- mackerel
- herring
- sardines
- anchovies
- canola oil
- flaxseed
- walnuts
- basil
- oregano
- sweet peppers

Cooling mint minimizes pain

Mint adds a refreshing zip to iced tea, fruit salad, and gum. But it may also provide a refreshing way to soothe arthritis pain.

Traditional Chinese healers used mint oil to treat injuries because of its anti-inflammatory powers and cooling effect on the skin, and ancient Greek doctors used cold-water compresses to ease swelling and joint pain.

Borrowing these tactics from ancient civilizations, University of Edinburgh researchers unveiled a synthetic treatment with the same cooling properties of mint oil. Their study suggests natural "minty" compounds can work just as well as more conventional painkillers — without addiction or side effects.

That's because they're applied directly to the skin, lessening the risk of adverse effects. Unlike morphine, for example, which is not always effective for chronic pain, this minty treatment should work on arthritis and nerve pain.

Move more to ache less

Every extra pound of body weight you carry puts the equivalent of 4 pounds of stress on your knees. So losing just a few pounds can make a big difference. Regular exercise can help you shed some of those extra pounds — and reduce the burden on your joints.

But exercise helps in other ways, too. In a mouse study, those fed a high-fat diet still saw improvements with exercise, even though they didn't lose weight. Somehow, exercise disrupted the inflammatory response to slow the development of arthritis.

Aerobic activities like swimming, cycling, and walking could do the same for you. Exercises that strengthen the muscles that support your joints or improve flexibility are especially helpful. Try yoga, tai chi, or stretching.

You may be sore at first. But in the long-run, you'll be rewarded with greater mobility and less pain.

Here's why. The compounds act through a pain receptor called TRPM8, which is found in some of your skin's nerve cells. When activated by the cooling chemicals or cool temperatures, TRPM8 shuts off the pain messages to your brain. So it enhances your body's natural painkilling mechanisms. This synthetic treatment combines the properties of mint oil with other elements that specifically target TRPM8.

Researchers hope to further develop these special mint compounds into a safe, effective treatment for chronic pain, including osteoarthritis. That means more tests and studies.

But in the meantime, you can soothe your arthritis pain like ancient doctors with a homemade cooling, minty salve. Just make sure to try it on a small patch of skin first to test for sensitivity.

This topical mint treatment proves that pain relief doesn't have to come with a prescription. Now that's refreshing.

Homemade minty salve

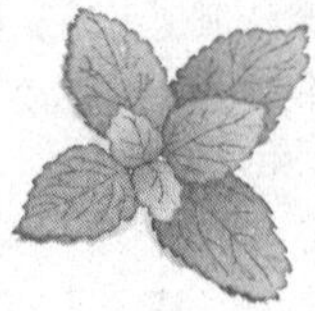

Take advantage of the pain-relieving properties of mint with this soothing salve. Here's what you'll need:

- 1 cup of olive oil
- 1-2 ounces of beeswax
- 1-2 drops of peppermint essential oil

Melt the olive oil and beeswax gently on low heat. Remove from heat and stir in the peppermint oil. Transfer the mixture to a clean container and let it cool completely. Store the container of salve in the refrigerator, where it should keep for up to a year.

Before applying the minty salve to your sore joints, make sure to try it on a small patch of skin to test for sensitivity. If all is well, rub it onto your skin, focusing on sore muscles and joints.

Hit a high 'C' to protect your knees

Could eating more papayas, strawberries, and oranges be the secret to pain-free knees for life? Research suggests it's a good bet if you eat foods like these that are loaded with vitamin C.

Australian researchers found that a high intake of this important vitamin reduced the risk of developing certain bone abnormalities that contribute to knee osteoarthritis (OA).

The study included 293 healthy, middle-aged people without knee osteoarthritis. Participants filled out food-frequency questionnaires to provide information on their diets. After approximately 10 years, they had MRIs on their knees to measure signs of degeneration, including cartilage volume, bone area, cartilage defects, and bone marrow lesions.

While vitamin C had no effect on cartilage, it did have positive effects on bone. Specifically, MRIs of people whose diets contained high levels of vitamin C showed reduced bone area and fewer bone marrow lesions.

That's important because both factors play a role in the development of knee osteoarthritis. Compared to people without OA, those with OA have increased bone area — and this area increases over time. Meanwhile, bone marrow lesions have been linked to pain and joint space loss in knee OA.

Although vitamin C is a powerful antioxidant, its beneficial effect on osteoarthritis is probably not due to its antioxidant powers. Rather, vitamin C likely helps because of its important role in bone health.

- Vitamin C is needed to form collagen, one of the building blocks of bone, ligaments, and tendons.
- It stimulates your body to make osteoblasts, or bone cells.
- It may also boost bone mineral density, a marker of bone strength.

Do your bones — and especially your knees — a favor and boost your vitamin C intake by eating these foods:

Fruits	Vegetables
papayas	peppers
strawberries	broccoli
raspberries	Brussels sprouts
pineapple	cauliflower
kiwifruit	cabbage
mango	kale
cantaloupe	collard greens
tangerines	tomatoes

Get 'hip' to garlic's protective powers

Hip hip hooray! Just by eating more garlic, you may lower your risk of osteoarthritis (OA) of the hip.

That's the good news from a King's College London study of more than 1,000 female twins.

- The study used food frequency questionnaires to track people's eating habits.
- There was an average follow-up of just over nine years.
- Researchers examined X-rays of participants' hands, hips, and knees to detect evidence of OA.

They discovered that women whose diets contained high levels of garlic and other allium vegetables — including onions, shallots, chives, and leeks — were less likely to develop hip osteoarthritis.

Surprisingly, no link was found between food intake and OA of the hand or knee. But this study suggests that you can protect your hips by changing your diet.

What makes garlic so powerful? Lab tests shed some light on how this herb may protect your joints. Diallyl disulphide, a compound found in garlic and other allium vegetables, represses the expression of matrix metalloproteinases (MMPs), enzymes that break down cartilage and contribute to osteoarthritis. But exactly how it keeps these enzymes in check remains a mystery. The compound's ability to act as an antioxidant or its anti-inflammatory powers could be the key.

However it works, garlic is a healthy — and flavorful — addition to your diet. While more research is needed to confirm and build on these promising results, you don't need to wait to mince, crush, chop, or grate some garlic into your favorite dishes.

Don't forget about the other allium vegetables, either. Onions, shallots, chives, and leeks can add flavor to any meal — while adding extra protection for your hips.

The diet secrets that will save your knees

Have you ever put bad gas in your car? It will run, but you won't get the best performance out of your engine. Your diet is not that different. If you eat the wrong foods, you run the risk of creating problems. Fortunately, these easy steps are all it takes to avoid filling up your body with the wrong fuel.

Need to curb your pain? Cut out carbs. You know that sweet drinks can spike your blood sugar, but did you know a can of soda could cause your knees to ache? How about a plate of mashed potatoes?

> High heels may look cute, but this fashion fad is a killer on your joints. Research says that wearing these types of shoes may contribute to the development of knee osteoarthritis.

Researchers studied how eating a diet rich in high-carb foods like potatoes, sodas, and white bread can affect your joints. They asked one group of seniors with knee osteoarthritis to stick with their normal diet, and instructed another group to eat a low-carb diet. After three months, the people who ate fewer carbs had less pain in their knees than those who didn't change the way they ate.

Scientists think this diet is so effective because it helps lower oxidative stress in your body, which in turn helps prevent pain in your joints. Plus an animal study revealed that diets high in sugar cause joint inflammation.

What does that mean for you? Instead of loading your plate with pasta and breadsticks, try eating more lean meats, fish, and vegetables.

Feast on fiber to dodge arthritis. You'll be happy to know that plant-based foods are loaded with fiber. Beans, legumes, and leafy greens are all outstanding sources of roughage. And that's great news for your joints.

A study of over 6,000 people found that those who ate the highest amount of fiber were much less likely to develop arthritis over a nine-year period than low-fiber eaters.

Changing diets by increasing intake of dietary fiber seems to be one of the most economic ways to reduce the risk of knee osteoarthritis," says Dr. Zhaoli Dai, lead author of the study.

If your diet is a little low on roughage, start by adding a bowl of oatmeal to your breakfast menu and snacking on more fruits and veggies. Dietary guidelines call for adults to eat 14 grams of fiber for every 1,000 calories each day.

And don't forget the beans and legumes. A single cup of cooked lentils clocks in at a whopping 15.6 grams of fiber.

Osteoporosis

Ward off frightening fractures

Half of all women and up to a quarter of men over age 50 will suffer a fracture triggered by osteoporosis. According to the National Osteoporosis Foundation, this disease caused more than 2 million fractures in one year alone. Those are scary statistics. Fortunately, research suggests you can help prevent these fractures by making sure you get enough vitamin D.

A review of studies found that people who get between 482 and 770 international units (IU) of vitamin D a day cut their hip fracture risk by 18 percent and reduce the odds of most other fractures by 20 percent. Although the people in the studies took supplements, you should aim to get as much vitamin D as possible from foods. That's because other nutrients in foods, like calcium, may further cut your odds of osteoporosis and fractures.

Build up your bones. Your skeleton gets remodeled just like the homes on HGTV. Every year, cells called osteoclasts clean out old bone, and cells called osteoblasts replace it with new. About 10% of your bones are replaced each year. Your body needs calcium and phosphorous from food to form new bone. It also needs collagen. Your body can make this nutrient, but you need vitamin C to do it. All these nutrients work together to build your bones and keep them strong.

Prevent bones from crumbling. Vitamin D has its own part to play. As you age, you start losing bone faster than you make it. That means your bones may gradually become full of holes like a sponge. Without enough calcium in your diet to help make new bone, your skeleton may break down even faster.

To absorb calcium from food, you need vitamin D, magnesium, and several other nutrients. But vitamin D may be particularly important. When you don't get enough vitamin D, you can only absorb 10 to 15 percent of the calcium in your food.

How Bone Remodeling Works

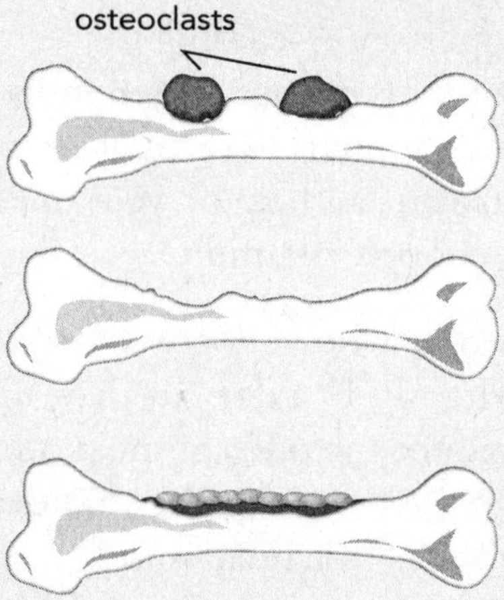

Bone-removing cells called osteoclasts release acids and enzymes that dissolve bone.

When they finish, the osteoclast cells disappear.

Bone-making cells called osteoblasts arrive.They lay down a framework of collagen and coat it with a mix of calcium and phosphorus.

When the osteoblasts finish, the bone is solid again — except when osteoclasts are removing bone faster than osteoblasts can make it. Then your bones have more holes, and your risk of osteoporosis goes up.

Pump up your vitamin D. Unfortunately, about 35% of adults in the United States are deficient in vitamin D. Current guidelines recommend that people age 70 and under get 600 international units (IU) of this important nutrient each day. Those age 71 and older should get 800 IU. So consider upping your vitamin D intake with these delicious choices.

Did you know?

Strong bones sound like your cup of tea? If so, feel free to drink up. Plant-based nutrients in tea — called polyphenols — can prevent or reverse damage to your cells by acting as antioxidants. And they may be responsible for keeping osteoporosis at bay.

Long-term tea drinkers have better bone density and bone strength than non-tea drinkers, according to several large studies. Experts believe it's all due to their polyphenols. So which type of tea is best for your bones?

You might want to opt for green tea. It contains several kinds of polyphenols that discourage the production of osteoclasts, the cells that break down bone tissue. Not only that, these compounds have also been found to increase the survival and growth of osteoblasts. Those are the cells that create bone tissue. Not a fan of green tea? Black tea polyphenols also support bone health. So have another cuppa!

- 400 or more IU — 3 ounces of cooked rainbow trout or wild-caught canned pink salmon. Mix the canned salmon with mustard and dill for a quick sandwich filling.
- 300 to 400 IU — a cup of chocolate malted drink mix stirred into 8 ounces of milk, or half a broiled or grilled halibut fillet.
- 100 to 300 IU — 8 ounces of soy milk with added vitamins, or 1 cup of fortified tofu.
- 50 to 100 IU — a cup of orange juice with added vitamin D, or a serving of some cereals and yogurts. Check labels for vitamin D content before buying.

Ask your doctor whether you should take vitamin D supplements and what dose you need.

Make smart choices to beat osteoporosis

Eat an entire cup of low-fat yogurt to start your day. Research suggests you need the calcium in that yogurt because most Americans over 50 don't get enough. It's a way to keep your bones strong at any age and protect against breaks.

Discover how deficiency sneaks in. Researchers from Yale University and the University of Connecticut examined the calcium and calorie intakes of more than 9,000 men and women. They discovered that people eat less calcium as they age. In fact, the amount of calcium most people get from food declines with each passing decade of life.

Part of the reason for this is that people tend to eat fewer calories as they age. As a result, older adults may eat smaller portions of calcium-rich foods or stop eating some food sources of calcium. This may not seem like a big deal, but the scientists found that study participants fell short of the daily recommended amount of calcium, even if they took supplements.

Choose a smarter solution. You might think the answer is to simply take a higher dose of supplements, but government dietary guidelines say it's better to get most nutrients from foods. Foods not only provide calcium but also supply fiber and bone-strengthening compounds you won't get from calcium pills.

> If you're having milk and calcium-fortified juice with your breakfast, take your calcium supplement at lunch or dinner. Your body can only absorb so much at one time.

This doesn't mean you should stop taking calcium supplements if your doctor recommends them. But you should also follow the advice of the Yale and Connecticut researchers, who recommend eating nutrient-dense foods, especially those that offer more calcium per serving.

To help reach the 1,200 milligrams (mg) of calcium recommended for women age 51 or older and men age 71 or older, switch to higher-calcium foods by making smart choices like these.

Extra calcium	by choosing	instead of
980 mg	1 cup of Total Raisin Bran 100% Nutrition (1000 mg)	1 cup of Kellogg's Raisin Bran (20 mg)
358 mg	8-ounce cup of low-fat fruit yogurt (372 mg)	1 blueberry muffin (14 mg)
348 mg	two slices of American cheese (356 mg)	3 ounces of roasted turkey breast (8 mg)
229 mg	3 ounces of pink canned salmon with bones (241 mg)	3 ounces of white tuna canned in water (12 mg)
129 mg	1 ounce of nonfat or fat-free mozzarella cheese (272 mg)	1 ounce of regular mozzarella cheese (143 mg)
83 mg	1/2 cup of boiled collard greens (134 mg)	1/2 cup of boiled Swiss chard (51 mg)

Go green for fracture-resistant bones

Leafy greens may be the number one food for keeping strong healthy bones if you don't like dairy foods, says Annemarie Colbin, author of *Food and Our Bones: The Natural Way to Prevent Osteoporosis.* Here are just a few of the advantages these greens offer.

- They come in many varieties, including collard greens, chicory, kale, mustard greens, parsley, spinach, turnip greens, watercress, and bok choy.
- Leafy greens are relatively inexpensive.
- Some experts say foods like meats and grains break down into acid byproducts in your body. Eating too many of those foods

HEALTH ALERT!

Ingredients in your diet can keep you from absorbing some or all of the calcium from foods. Watch out for these when planning your menu.

- Wheat bran. A food that's 100 percent wheat bran may limit the calcium you absorb from other foods you eat with it.
- Salt. Research suggests that eating more than 1 teaspoon of salt a day can increase the amount of calcium you lose. Fortunately, eating seven or eight servings of potassium-rich foods like potatoes, dates, raisins, and tomato sauce can help you lose less calcium. So can cutting back on salt.
- Oxalates. The natural compound oxalate occurs in foods like cranberries, chard, spinach, and dried beans. Oxalate binds up the calcium in these foods so you cannot absorb most of it. These foods have other nutrients you need, so don't stop eating them. Just depend on other foods for calcium, instead.

may trigger a process that pulls calcium from your bones. But leafy greens may produce alkaline byproducts during digestion. That may help protect your bones from acids.

- These foods supply your body with calcium, potassium, and other nutrients you need to make new bone — including vitamin K.

In fact, leafy greens are a leading source of vitamin K. You need this vitamin because you constantly dispose of old bone and replace it with new bone. Vitamin K contributes to osteocalcin, a key protein needed for new bone.

If you have a vitamin K deficiency, your body forms a less effective version of osteocalcin that is commonly found in people with osteoporosis. But if you take in enough vitamin K, your body makes high-quality osteocalcin that helps weave new bone into a fracture-resistant pattern. This may be one reason why studies suggest vitamin K supplements may reduce bone and calcium loss. It may also help explain why research links low vitamin K intake to poorer bone mineral density and an increased risk of fractures.

Even mild vitamin K deficiency may threaten your bones, researchers suspect. They point out that vitamin K is required by one set of proteins that help your blood clot, but it is also required by other vital proteins, including the osteocalcin in bone.

Animal research suggests your body rations vitamin K when you don't take in enough of it. First, your body provides enough vitamin K for the proteins that coagulate your blood. Then, if any is left, your body supplies vitamin K for other proteins like osteocalcin. So if you don't get enough of this nutrient, you may constantly form new bone with second-rate osteocalcin. And that may put you at higher risk for osteoporosis and future fractures.

Of course, you may avoid this problem by eating plenty of leafy greens. A good way to sneak them in is to add finely chopped kale, spinach, or bok choy to soups, casseroles, stews, chili, stir-fries, or marinara sauce. But if you take a blood-thinning drug like warfarin, talk to your doctor before adding more vitamin K to your diet. Vitamin K can make blood-thinning medications less effective.

Crispy kale chips

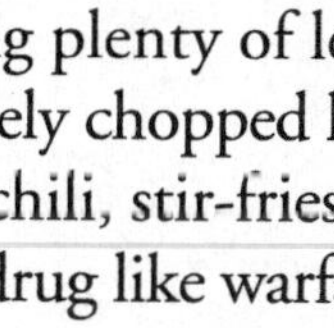

Make your own kale chips. Wash and dry the kale, remove the center rib, and tear the leaves into chip-size pieces. Toss these with salt, olive oil, and lemon juice, spread them in a single layer on a pan, and bake at 300 degrees about 20 to 25 minutes, until crispy.

Strengthen your skeleton with prunes

Meet the next superfood of the fruit world. You're bound to love the sweet flavor. And researchers are surprised at just how much disease-fighting power prunes have — especially against the brittle-bone disease osteoporosis. You can eat figs, apples, dates, strawberries, or raisins, and you still won't get the same bone-boosting results women have already gotten from prunes.

Researchers even put this to the test. They asked one group of women to eat prunes every day for a year while another group ate dried apples. Both groups took a daily 500-milligram calcium supplement and a 400-international-unit vitamin D supplement.

The study found that the women who ate 10 prunes a day showed improvement in the bone mineral density of their spines and wrists compared to the dried apple eaters. That's important because bone mineral density shows how strong your bones are. The density of your spine and wrist can be particularly critical because osteoporosis-caused fractures often happen in those bones.

Did you know?

Prunes contain oxalates, the compound that binds with calcium and prevents your body from absorbing it. But don't fret. The oxalates in prunes can only prevent you from absorbing calcium from the fruit itself. Your body can still take in calcium from any other foods you eat with prunes. So if you dice this fruit and mix it into yogurt, you won't miss out on any of yogurt's valuable calcium. And you'll still benefit from the polyphenols and other nutrients in prunes.

But that's not all the researchers learned. The prune eaters also had lower levels of two indicator compounds that drop when your bone loss slows down. This means that prunes may help you lose less bone.

Evidence continues to build supporting the theory that powerful compounds in prunes called polyphenols play an important role in combating bone loss. This fruit is also a good source of nutrients like vitamin K, potassium, and boron, which may also play a key role in protecting your skeleton.

Try adding finely chopped prunes to rice pilaf, chicken salad, or trail mix. Or stir them into your oatmeal or yogurt. In fact, you can even substitute finely chopped prunes for raisins in muffins and other baked goods. The California Prune Board also recommends these ideas:

- Add pitted finely chopped prunes to peanut butter for a satisfying spread for toast or bagels.
- Dip whole pitted prunes in melted dark chocolate. Let them harden on wax paper before you try this tasty treat.
- Tuck an almond inside a pitted prune for a sweet, crunchy, and healthy snack.

Super snack beats brittle bones

Don't throw away those pumpkin seeds when you carve your jack-o-lantern. You can turn them into sweet treats, garlic-flavored nibbles, or spicy snacks quickly and easily. And because pumpkin seeds are rich in magnesium, they can help fend off magnesium deficiencies that are more common in women than men. That's important because studies suggest you need more of this mineral to protect your bones.

- Magnesium helps stimulate cells and enzymes that your body needs to maintain a healthy skeleton. Animal studies suggest that not getting enough of it could cause a decrease in bone mineral density, leading to osteoporosis.
- Low blood levels of magnesium may lead to low blood levels of calcium and vitamin D, plus have other effects. This may result in less new bone formation and more bone loss.
- The less magnesium in your bones, the bigger bone crystals grow as they form. This makes bone more fragile. And, in fact, some studies have found that women with osteoporosis have less magnesium in their bones and larger bone crystals than women who don't have osteoporosis.

Older adults tend to have less magnesium in their diet than younger adults. What's more, your gut absorbs less magnesium as you get older. And your aging kidneys excrete more of this nutrient. Aim for a magnesium-rich diet to hit your daily recommended amount of 320 milligrams (mg) for women and 420 mg for men.

To add more magnesium to your menu, sprinkle unsalted pumpkin seeds on salads or hot or cold cereals. You can also add them to a stir-fry, or blend them in a trail mix. For a tempting snack, roast the seeds from your Halloween pumpkin. Here's how.

- Drop the seeds in a bowl of water. Rapidly rub them with your hands to remove most of the pulp.
- Spray a cookie sheet with vegetable oil, and spread the seeds in a single layer on the sheet.
- Lightly spray over the seeds with vegetable oil, and sprinkle a topping on them. Try cinnamon and pumpkin pie spice for a sweet taste, cayenne pepper and thyme for a spicier bite, or just use garlic powder.

- Roast the seeds for 15 minutes at 175 degrees, let cool, and enjoy this tasty snack.

Just be sure to limit yourself to one handful of pumpkin seeds a day, so you won't gain weight.

For more magnesium, enjoy foods like black beans, white beans, Brazil nuts, baby lima beans, black-eyed peas, oat bran muffins, and boiled, chopped spinach.

HEALTH ALERT!

Check the labels of any antacids, laxatives, calcium supplements, or other medications and supplements you take regularly. If these contain magnesium, be careful not to take too much. An overdose of magnesium can cause diarrhea and potentially dangerous magnesium toxicity.

But don't let your magnesium levels drop too low, either. Long-term use of a family of drugs called proton pump inhibitors (PPIs) can lower your magnesium levels. PPIs typically help treat problems like gastroesophageal reflux disease (GERD) and ulcers.

Low blood levels of magnesium may cause no symptoms, or they may lead to serious problems like dangerous muscle spasms, irregular heartbeat, or convulsions. If you take a PPI, talk to your doctor about your magnesium levels — especially if you also take medications like digoxin, diuretics, or other drugs that may lower magnesium. PPIs may cause dangerous interactions when taken with medications like these.

Ancient spice fends off bone loss

An ancient spice found in modern mustard may help keep your bones strong, research suggests. Turmeric has long been popular in India, China, and Indonesia, but now you have a special reason to add this pungent, golden-orange spice to your spice rack.

Bone loss speeds up after menopause. So a study from the University of Arizona tried turmeric to slow the bone loss of animals that had experienced the equivalent of menopause. The researchers tested two turmeric extracts similar to the turmeric supplements available to consumers. Both extracts contained curcuminoids — powerful natural compounds that may limit your body's population of bone-removing osteoclast cells. Fewer osteoclasts may mean less bone loss.

HEALTH ALERT!

Losing three-fourths of an inch of height between ages 40 and 70 is not unusual for a woman. But researchers found a significantly higher risk of hip fracture in both men and women over age 70 who lost 2 inches or more in two years.

Experts now say height loss can serve as an early warning system for osteoporosis. So start tracking your height, no matter what your age. Ask to have your height measured at your next doctor's visit, and get a new measurement every year.

Meanwhile, take steps to prevent or slow height loss, such as getting plenty of calcium and vitamin D, eating a healthy diet, and participating in regular weight-bearing exercises like walking or gardening.

Curcuminoids made up only 41 percent of extract A, while they made up 94 percent of extract B. As a result, extract A did not have much effect, but extract B made a difference in three ways.

- Animals who received extract B three times a week lost up to 50 percent less bone density than animals that didn't.
- Extract B helped protect trabecular bone, the kind in the hip and other common sites of fractures caused by osteoporosis.
- Extract B helped prevent damage to their bones' internal structure and other bone characteristics that help determine how strong your bones are. This may make bones more resistant to fractures.

More studies are needed, of course, but early research suggests that turmeric can also help humans in the fight against osteoporosis. The scientists, meanwhile, say they need to establish which turmeric supplements contain the right curcuminoids in the right amounts.

So you'll want to add more turmeric to your diet. Although the extracts in the study are far more powerful than dried turmeric root, the dried root contains essential oils you won't find in the extracts or in turmeric supplements. The oils help you absorb a higher percentage of the curcuminoids in foods.

Turmeric's flavor does not appeal to everyone. Adding small amounts to foods that mask the taste is an easy way to enjoy its benefits.

You can start by adding a 1/4 teaspoon of turmeric to chili, hot chocolate, hot milk, ketchup, pasta sauce, mustard, soups, stews, tomato juice, curry, or to vegetables as you sauté them. You can increase the amount to 1/2 teaspoon or 1 teaspoon depending on your taste.

Just be sure to talk to your doctor before you add more turmeric to your diet. Turmeric may be unsafe for people with gallstones, ulcers, and several other health conditions.

Hidden benefit of cheese

Cheese tends to be high in calories, so many dieters put it on their forbidden food list. But it can actually be good for your health. Not only are many cheeses a great source of calcium, they also contain a skeleton-saving nutrient called conjugated linoleic acid (CLA).

A University of Connecticut study examined the diets and bone density of women who had already experienced menopause. They discovered that women who ate more CLA had better bone density in the forearm, a common place for osteoporosis fractures. The scientists also found a link between CLA and the bone density of Ward's triangle, an area of bone in the hip.

Experts suspect CLA lowers the amount of prostaglandin E2 (PGE2) in your bones. That's good news because too much PGE2 may hamper your bone-making cells, called osteoblasts, and reduce the amount of new bone they make. Because older women lose bone faster than they make it, PGE2 can contribute to substantial bone loss. But lower levels of this prostaglandin may encourage your body to generate more new bone.

To add more CLA to your diet, include dairy products in your daily menu. Full-fat brick cheese provides 7.1 milligrams (mg) of CLA in each gram of fat. That's nearly 57 grams of CLA in 1 ounce. Here's how much CLA you can get from an ounce of other full-fat cheeses.

- muenster – 56 grams
- colby – 54.9 grams
- cheddar – 38.5 grams
- mozzarella – 30.8 grams
- ricotta – 22.4 grams
- cottage – 4.5 grams

Of course, government dietary guidelines recommend you eat low-fat versions of dairy foods and limit yourself to three servings each day. Less fat in cheeses may mean less CLA. If you're concerned, try eating reduced-fat Swiss cheese. For some reason, this one goes against the norm, giving you 14 mg of CLA in 1.5 ounces. For even better results, try these smart tactics.

Eat Pecorino-Romano. A study suggests Pecorino-Romano cheese made from sheep's milk has three to five times as much CLA as regular cow's milk cheeses like cheddar. Although it is not low in fat, dieters use this cheese to flavor foods because a little goes a long way — plus it's a great substitute for Parmesan cheese. Look for the sheep's head logo to make sure you buy cheese made from the milk of grass-fed sheep. That grass-fed diet makes Pecorino-Romano much richer in CLA.

Choose grass-fed, low-fat dairy. Check your supermarket's cheese and deli sections for other cheeses from grass-fed cows. Most cattle are fed grains instead of grass, and that lowers the CLA content in their milk. But research shows that cows fed exclusively on pasture grass may produce up to 500 percent more CLA in milk than cows fed a typical dairy farm diet. That may mean more CLA in low-fat cheese.

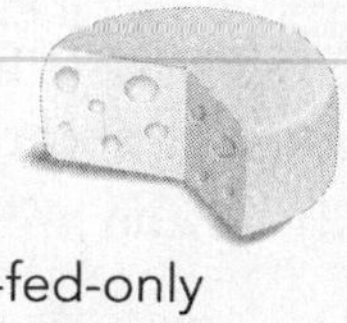

Meat or cheese labeled "grass fed" may still come from a cow that has been fed grain products or given hormones and antibiotics. To make sure the product comes from grass-fed-only cattle with higher amounts of conjugated linoleic acid (CLA), look for one of these labels instead.

- 100 percent grass fed. This means the animal was not fed any grain or grain byproducts. These animals usually are not given hormones or antibiotics either.
- American Grassfed Association (AGA) label. The AGA label indicates the animal has been fed a diet of grass and hay and has not been confined in a pen or given hormones or antibiotics.

Enjoy a little beef. Try an occasional 5-ounce serving of lamb, veal, or lean fresh ground beef or ground round. These foods are also good sources of CLA. Choose grass-fed meat if your budget allows.

Consider a supplement. Ask your doctor about CLA supplements if you think you can't get enough from foods.

Go fishing for bone-boosting fats

You already know salmon is good for your heart, but research suggests it's good for your bones, too. After examining the diets and hipbones of more than 600 older adults, researchers found that those who ate three or more servings of fish each week fared better. But which fish you choose and whether you're a man or a woman makes a big difference.

Dark fish are cold-water, fatty fish like salmon, bluefish, or sardines, which are high in omega-3 fatty acids like docosahexaenoic acid (DHA) and eicosapentaenoic acid (EPA.) Men who regularly ate dark fish, tuna, or both lost less bone in the femoral neck hipbone over a four-year period. That's important because the femoral neck is prone to fractures. The researchers also found that the more of these fish men ate, the less bone they lost.

But tuna did not help women. Instead, over a four-year period, women who ate the most servings of dark fish each week lost little or no bone from the femoral neck compared with women who ate fewer servings.

The scientists behind the study could not pin down exactly how eating fish may help protect your bones, but they suggest several possibilities.

- The EPA and DHA in fish may help your body keep more calcium and move it to your bones.
- Omega-3 fatty acids may help control the compound prostaglandin E2, which promotes bone loss at high levels. Omega-3 may also help produce bone-creating cells and play a role in creating other compounds that help prevent bone loss.
- High levels of the omega-6 fatty acid linoleic acid (LA) were linked to more bone loss in women participating in the study. At least one other study suggests you're more likely to lose bone if you eat more omega-6 fatty acids than omega-3. But fish — especially dark fish — usually have a higher ratio of omega-3 fatty acids, which may protect you against LA's effects.

Antlers reveal a new cause of osteoporosis

Deer antlers, like human bones, need a good calcium supply. But when fragile, broken deer antlers became widespread in Spain, the deer had plenty of calcium in their diets. Instead, a harsh winter had kept them from getting enough manganese. That led Spanish scientists to suspect you need manganese to prevent calcium loss.

Manganese also supports crucial organs like your brain. If you don't get enough, your body may pull manganese from your bones to keep your brain or other vital organs going. Without enough manganese in your skeleton, your bones may not be able to absorb all the calcium they need. Over time, that loss could weaken your skeleton and eventually lead to osteoporosis.

More studies are needed to determine whether a manganese shortage actually causes osteoporosis. So keep your eyes peeled for future developments.

Here's a quick way to get more fish into your diet. Buy one 6-ounce can of wild-caught pink salmon. Mash up the fish. For a delicious Mexican sandwich filling, stir in a 1/4 cup of salsa. Or if you're looking for a tasty Italian sandwich filling, stir in 2 tablespoons of low-fat or fat-free Italian dressing with a sprinkle of oregano or basil.

Juicy red bone-builder you should eat every day

Women who regularly enjoy tomato juice, pasta sauces, and raw tomatoes may lose bone more slowly that those who don't eat tomatoes or tomato products, a Canadian study reports. So if you're a tomato lover, eat up.

Scientists recruited women ages 50 to 60 and checked their blood for lycopene levels and signs of bone loss. Lycopene is the pigment that helps turn tomatoes and watermelon red. Scientists think you may also need it to help protect your bones.

To find out, the researchers asked the women to avoid tomatoes, tomato products, and any other foods that contained lycopene for one month. When the month ended, the lycopene levels in the women's blood had dropped, but they had higher blood levels of N-telopeptide (NTx), a compound that increases as bone loss speeds up.

> If you avoid nightshade vegetables like tomatoes due to concerns about arthritis, ask your doctor if you should take lycopene supplements.

The researchers concluded the absence of lycopene may have contributed to bone loss, but they wondered if regular doses of lycopene would also help prevent bone loss. In their next study, they asked 60 women between ages 50 and 60 to avoid lycopene for a month. At the end of the month, they divided the women into four groups.

- Group 1 drank tomato juice with 30 milligrams (mg) of lycopene daily.
- Group 2 drank tomato juice with 70 mg of lycopene each day.
- Group 3 took 30 mg of lycopene daily.
- Group 4 took a placebo supplement.

After four months, the women who drank tomato juice or took lycopene had significantly higher lycopene levels and lower NTx levels in their blood than the women who took a placebo. So the scientists concluded lycopene may help prevent bone loss.

Lycopene may help because it has antioxidant powers to help fight free radical damage. Free radicals are broken molecules that occur throughout your body. They repair themselves by stealing electrons from cells, but this can leave the cells permanently damaged.

Scientists call this damage oxidation. Antioxidants prevent oxidation by donating electrons to the free radical before it can steal from a cell. That is good news because free radicals may promote bone loss by causing your body to make more bone-removing cells and fewer bone-making cells. And in fact, research suggests free radicals speed up bone loss.

Fortunately, the Canadian researchers found that the women who drank or took lycopene regularly had lower levels of oxidation and a higher capacity to prevent oxidation than the women who took placebo capsules. Less oxidation may mean less bone loss and lower odds of osteoporosis.

Just 30 mg of lycopene a day was enough to help the women in the study. You can easily get that from a cup of canned tomato sauce or ready-to-eat marinara sauce, or 11 ounces of canned tomato juice or vegetable juice cocktail.

Did you know?

Mom always said you should eat all your vegetables. Now experts suspect your bones may depend on it. Here's their theory. When your body digests cereal grains, dairy foods, and meats, they break down into acids that raise the acidity of your blood. Your body may draw calcium from your bones to help neutralize these acids.

But when you eat fruits and vegetables, they break down into alkaline compounds, which may help neutralize excess acids in your bloodstream. What's more, many fruits and vegetables are high in potassium, vitamin C, and other nutrients that play key roles in defending your bones. So aim for four to five daily servings of both fruits and vegetables like apricots, spinach, kiwifruit, zucchini, carrots, oranges, raisins, and tomatoes.

Ovarian cancer

Cut out cold cuts to lower risk

Ovarian cancer is a relatively rare form of cancer, yet it is the fifth-leading cause of cancer death among women in the United States. Even worse, many cases aren't found until it's too late.

But there's good news. Researchers in Australia found that you can cut your risk of ovarian cancer by substituting fish or poultry for the processed meats on your plate. That means aiming to eat more salmon and tuna and less salami and hot dogs.

The researchers looked at two studies that analyzed what women ate and who got ovarian cancer. Overall, eating more meat did not affect their risk. But women who ate the most processed meats showed a higher risk of developing ovarian cancer, while those who ate the most fish and poultry had a lower risk. Eating fish at least four times a week offered the greatest protection.

The reason for these results is unclear. But many processed meats contain nitrites and nitrates, which can form nitrosamines — known carcinogens for animals. In addition, fish contains healthy omega-3 fatty acids, believed to protect your cells.

Other research found that women who ate more red meat, processed meat, eggs, butter and margarine, and desserts like cake, candy, and cookies had a higher risk of developing ovarian cancer.

So replace meats — especially processed meats — with fish to lower your risk of this deadly cancer. Try these tricks to put more fish and poultry on your plate.

- Leave the steaks at the store, and bring home salmon instead. It will be great on the grill.
- Enjoy soft tacos made with grilled cod rather than beef.
- Use ground chicken or turkey in your chili in place of hamburger.
- Drizzle olive oil, garlic, and spices on fish or boneless chicken, then broil it in the oven until it's cooked thoroughly. You won't miss that sausage.

Sunshine vitamin pumps up protection

You may be able to prevent ovarian cancer with a surprising nutrient — vitamin D. A lack of the sunshine vitamin has been linked to ovarian cancer risk, adding to the list of other ailments this hard-working vitamin may fight.

Experts noticed that women in parts of the world that don't get a lot of sun were more likely to develop ovarian cancer. You get a lot of your vitamin D supply from sun exposure, so they wanted to see if there was a link.

The researchers looked at a group of U.S. women, some with and some without ovarian cancer. Women who had been ill with ovarian cancer were more than three times likely to have low levels of vitamin D in their blood. When researchers took into consideration age and the amount of calcium in the women's diets, they found that those with cancer were four times more likely to be vitamin D deficient.

Many older adults don't get enough vitamin D. Fortunately, your doctor can check the levels of this nutrient in your blood with a simple test. He may recommend lifestyle changes or help you find the right supplement.

Cut your cancer risk with strawberries

Want to get a head start on cancer prevention? Strawberries are the first fruits to ripen in the spring. Add in their track record for crimping cancer, and you have a yummy first line of defense.

Strawberries get their kick from flavonoids. These plant compounds are the stars of a study published in *The American Journal of Clinical Nutrition.* Researchers recruited more than 1,000 women over the age of 75 and followed them for five years. They recorded 73 percent fewer cancer deaths in ladies who ate the most flavonoids compared to those who ate the least.

Experts think that the compounds in strawberries may lower your risk for ovarian, bone, esophageal, and colon cancers.

3 drinks help sidestep cancer

Whether you prefer coffee, black tea, or green tea in the morning, you're doing your body good. Research suggests that all three of these beverages can cut the risk of certain cancers.

Green tea's EGCG hits tumors hard. That little polyphenol with the big name, epigallocatechin-3-gallate (EGCG), is believed to prevent cancer. Various studies have suggested it may keep at bay tumors of the prostate, lungs, colon, and breast.

Green tea is loaded with EGCG, so researchers in Sweden included it on a list of beverages and foods to see what might protect women against ovarian cancer. They surveyed more than 61,000 women who were middle-aged and older.

Women who drank tea, whether green or black, were less likely to develop ovarian cancer over the 15 years of the study. For every additional cup of tea a woman drank daily, she was about 18 percent less likely to develop this type of cancer.

Black tea gives a nutritional boost. Researchers in Australia studied a group of 2,700 women, half of whom had been ill with ovarian cancer. After looking at the differences in their eating habits, the researchers concluded that those who drank 4 or more cups of tea daily — whether black or green tea — cut their risk of ovarian cancer by nearly one-third. Tea is naturally high in protective antioxidants.

Other research focusing on black tea has shown that drinking as little as two cups daily might cut your risk of ovarian cancer.

Coffee puts the brakes on endometrial cancer. Because coffee can affect insulin and estrogen, two hormones related to cancer of the endometrium, or uterus lining, researchers wanted to see if coffee drinkers had a lower risk. They looked at information from the Nurses' Health Study, covering 67,470 women.

Women who drank 4 or more cups of coffee every day had a 25 percent lower risk of developing endometrial cancer over the 26 years of the study. Women who drank decaffeinated coffee were also protected, but not as much. So the researchers believe caffeine may be the main defense.

HEALTH ALERT!

Put down the potato chips. Older women who eat more high-acrylamide foods, including potato chips, french fries, and baked goods, have a higher risk of developing ovarian and endometrial cancer.

Acrylamides are natural compounds formed in high-carbohydrate foods during the baking, browning, and frying processes. Other studies also found higher risks among women in the Netherlands who ate more high-acrylamide cakes.

If cake, fries, or potato chips are your favorite snack, save them for a rare treat. Your ovaries will thank you.

Pancreatic cancer

Fabulous foods that fight back

Put the right foods on your plate, and you might protect yourself from pancreatic cancer. Promising research suggests that diet may play a role in fighting this deadly disease.

Pancreatic cancer can be a lethal enemy. Although it's a relatively uncommon disease, it has a five-year survival rate of only about 13 percent. With no early symptoms, it often goes undetected until it has progressed to a late stage.

Besides family history of the disease, potential risk factors include obesity, smoking, and diabetes. Standard treatment involves chemotherapy, radiation, or a combination of the two. Surgery and targeted therapy are other options.

Fortunately, you could reduce your risk of getting pancreatic cancer by turning to nature's remedies. Try these powerful food choices to keep this type of cancer at bay.

Gobble more grapes. The skins of red grapes contain a compound called resveratrol that may be a weapon against pancreatic cancer. In lab tests, resveratrol triggers apoptosis, or cell death, in pancreatic cancer cells. It seems to work by disrupting the function of the cancer cells' mitochondria, or energy centers. Other sources of resveratrol include blueberries, raspberries, peanuts, and red wine.

Pick out some produce. A Mayo Clinic study suggests that a diet rich in fruits and vegetables — as well as fiber and whole grains — may lessen your risk of developing pancreatic cancer. Specifically, citrus fruits, melons, berries, orange and grapefruit juice, dark green vegetables, deep yellow vegetables, and dry beans and peas provided protection.

Boost your B vitamins. Studies have found that people who get a lot of vitamin B6, vitamin B12, and folate from food sources — but not from supplements — may lower their risk of pancreatic cancer. Folate-rich foods include green leafy vegetables, cruciferous vegetables, oranges, legumes, and whole grains. You can find vitamin B6 in dark leafy greens, seafood, legumes, whole grains, fruits, and veggies. Meats, fish, dairy products, and eggs provide vitamin B12.

Treat yourself to tomatoes. A Canadian study found that a diet rich in lycopene, a carotenoid found mainly in tomatoes, could lower men's risk of pancreatic cancer by 31 percent. Guava, papaya, pink grapefruit, and watermelon also contain lycopene.

Did you know?

Once upon a time, coffee was thought to increase your risk of developing pancreatic cancer. But the opposite may be true. An analysis of 14 studies from the United States, Europe, and Japan suggests that drinking coffee actually lowers your risk.

Overall, regular coffee drinkers reduced their risk of developing pancreatic cancer by 18 percent compared to people who never or rarely drank coffee. Low to moderate coffee drinkers saw their risk decline by 14 percent, while heavy coffee drinkers slashed their risk by 32 percent. Just boosting your coffee intake by a cup a day may lead to a 4 percent reduction in pancreatic cancer risk.

More research is needed to confirm these findings, but brewing a pot of coffee could be an easy way to bolster your defenses against pancreatic cancer.

Minimize little-known meat risks

It's hard to beat burgers or steaks on the grill. But if you like your meat well-done, you may be increasing your risk of pancreatic cancer. In fact, meat itself — no matter how it's cooked — may boost your risk. Discover the potential dangers and how you can protect yourself.

Heterocyclic amines spell trouble. One study of more than 62,000 people found that those who liked their steak well-done had a 60 percent greater risk of developing pancreatic cancer compared to those who preferred rarer steaks or didn't eat steak at all.

Shed those extra pounds, and you may also drop your risk for pancreatic cancer. The American Cancer Society says being obese raises the risk of developing pancreatic cancer by 20 percent.

Chemicals called heterocyclic amines (HCAs) are likely to blame. These compounds are formed when animal protein is exposed to high temperatures for a long time. HCAs have been linked to a variety of cancers, including pancreatic, colon, breast, stomach, lung, and prostate cancers.

A Swedish analysis of 11 studies suggested that processed and red meat may boost your risk of pancreatic cancer. Another study found that those who ate the most saturated fat from animal food sources, including red meat, increased their risk of pancreatic cancer by 43 percent compared to those whose diets contained the least.

Grilling guidelines. Consider cutting back on meat — especially processed meats like hot dogs, bacon, and sausage — and making vegetables a larger part of each meal. But if you can't resist your carnivorous cravings, take these steps to make your meaty meals safer.

- Marinate your meat. A simple marinade, with acidic components like lemon juice or vinegar, can reduce HCAs by as much as 96 percent.
- Spice it up. Spices like rosemary and turmeric do more than add flavor to meat dishes. Their antioxidant powers also help prevent HCAs from forming.
- Cool it. Sear your meat, then move it to a cooler part of the grill to finish cooking under indirect heat. Raising the grill rack and flipping your meat often also helps.
- Decrease doneness. Opt for rare, medium-rare, or medium steaks to cut your cancer risk. To guard against undercooking, use a meat thermometer.

HEALTH ALERT!

Sipping sugary soft drinks could have some bitter consequences. The Singapore Chinese Health Study, which followed more than 60,000 participants for up to 14 years, found that people who drank two or more sugar-sweetened carbonated beverages a week boosted their risk of developing pancreatic cancer by 87 percent compared to those who drank none.

It's not just sugary drinks you need to worry about. Beware of a diet rich in foods that rank high on the Glycemic Index (GI), which measures how quickly a food causes your blood sugar to rise. An Italian study found that sweet, refined carbohydrates like sugar, candy, honey, and jam — all high-GI foods — elevated the risk of pancreatic cancer.

What makes these sugary foods so dangerous? UCLA researchers discovered that pancreatic cancer cells can grow by using fructose as fuel. The main source of this refined sugar is high-fructose corn syrup, a sweetener added to many foods and beverages, including soft drinks.

Parkinson's disease

Berries offer vital protection

The stakes have gotten higher when it comes to healthy eating. Research from Japan shows that people who eat lots of fruits, vegetables, mushrooms, seaweed, and fish have a lower risk of developing Parkinson's disease (PD) than those who eat a more typical Western diet, with lots of meat, sugar, and processed foods.

Berries are especially beneficial. Other researchers found that boosting berry intake may give even more Parkinson's protection. In a study that followed people for up to 22 years, men who ate the most high-flavonoid foods like blueberries and blackberries had a 40 percent lower risk of developing PD than men who ate the least.

Anthocyanins, colorful natural plant chemicals in blueberries, cranberries, and blackberries, are the class of flavonoids credited for the protection. Women in the study who ate the most anthocyanins also showed some protection against PD, although their overall consumption of flavonoids didn't make much difference.

> Anthocyanins are the natural plant chemicals that make blood oranges bright red inside. Common in many fruits, like blueberries and cranberries, anthocyanins are unusual in citrus fruits.

Anthocyanins and other flavonoids seem to help nerve cells handle stress and avoid damage, possibly due to their antioxidant power. So fill your plate with 3 cups of berries each week, plus lots of veggies and fish, and keep your hands tremor-free as you age.

HEALTH ALERT!

There's no single test to find out if you have Parkinson's disease, but early signs of the condition include tremors in a hand or leg, stiffness in your limbs, changes in handwriting, a weakened sense of smell, and difficulty sleeping due to thrashing around.

Parkinson's can also make it hard to swallow food, sometimes leading to unwanted weight loss. Try these tricks to help dinner go down smoothly.

- Sit comfortably upright at the table while you eat.
- Take small bites.
- Sip water before and during a meal to make chewing and swallowing easier.
- Replace thin, watery soups with thicker, creamy soups.
- Skip hard-to-swallow bread, and eat noodles or mashed potatoes instead.
- Enjoy meat with gravy or sauce for easier chewing.

Go nuts for healthy nerves

Feed pecans to mice doomed to develop Lou Gehrig's disease, and they stay healthy longer. That's what researchers found when they tested a nutty diet on mice bred to develop the condition, also known as amyotrophic lateral sclerosis (ALS). This finding is important for people looking to avoid another condition that affects your nerves — Parkinson's disease.

The high level of vitamin E in pecans and other nuts may help keep your nerves healthy. Experts say this powerful antioxidant may protect against age-related motor neuron degeneration — the cell damage responsible for conditions like Parkinson's disease and Alzheimer's disease.

One ounce of pecans has 0.40 milligrams (mg) of vitamin E. That's good, but you can do even better if vitamin E is what you're after. How about getting 1.6 mg of the vitamin from eating an ounce of Brazil nuts, or a whopping 7.3 mg from an ounce of almonds?

Aside from their vitamin E content, pecans are the tree nut that's highest in overall antioxidant power. Plus they're just so delicious.

Pecans and other nuts are high in calories, no matter how healthy they are. Fit them into your diet with a little attention to portion control. One ounce of pecans, which provides 196 calories, is about 19 pecan halves.

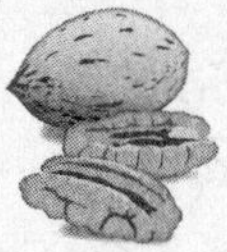

Two-way protection from fish

A fish dinner, like broiled tuna, cod, or salmon, is loaded with vitamins for your brain. These cold water fish are teeming with vitamin B6 and vitamin D — just what you need to get protection from Parkinson's disease in two important ways.

Vitamin B6 keeps homocysteine at bay. Researchers in Japan found that people with low levels of vitamin B6 had a roughly 50 percent higher risk of developing Parkinson's disease. The researchers compared people with Parkinson's with people who had no problems with a loss of nerve cells. Interestingly, other water-soluble vitamins, including vitamin B12, folate, and riboflavin, were not related to Parkinson's risk.

Experts think the power of vitamin B6 is its ability to bring down blood levels of homocysteine, an amino acid that can damage brain cells.

One cup of oil-packed light tuna provides nearly 50 percent of the vitamin D you need in a day, while the same serving of water-packed light tuna has basically none.

Vitamin D protects your nerves. Researchers in Finland followed a group of middle-aged and older folks for 29 years, checking their vitamin D levels and tracking who developed Parkinson's disease. Turns out people with the highest levels of vitamin D were 67 percent less likely to develop Parkinson's disease than those with the lowest levels.

Vitamin D may protect your brain because it works as an antioxidant, regulates calcium in your body, and helps conduct electricity through your body's nervous system.

For more information about eating fish to boost vitamin D in your diet, see "D-fend yourself from frightening fractures" in the *Osteoporosis* chapter.

Help from a surprising source

Drinking up to 4 cups of coffee daily may block damage to your brain from conditions like Parkinson's disease and Alzheimer's disease.

Researchers looked back at 26 studies on caffeine, coffee drinking, and Parkinson's to look at their connection. Overall, the studies found consuming caffeine from coffee and other foods cut the risk of developing Parkinson's by up to 25 percent.

Experts have considered several possible reasons caffeine may protect your nervous system. One idea is that it helps by attaching to certain receptors in the brain, blocking the natural chemical adenosine. In people with Parkinson's disease, adenosine slows down brain activity in the striatum, bringing on symptoms. Another possibility is that caffeine beefs up the blood brain barrier, helping protect your brain from toxins.

No matter the reason, you can enjoy your morning cup of Joe knowing you may be defending your brain.

Prostate cancer

Stymie cancer with broccoli

Want to live longer? Eat broccoli. This cruciferous vegetable contains a specific nutrient that literally switches on immunity-boosting disease fighters in your body, keeping you healthier as you age. Broccoli's secret weapon is sulforaphane, a phytochemical that fights cancer in a variety of ways.

Strengthens your immune system. A University of California, Los Angeles, study of mice found that sulforaphane activates an important protein called Nrf2, which regulates more than 200 antioxidant and protective genes as part of the immune response. For some reason, aging leads to a decrease in Nrf2 activity and a weakened immune system. But sulforaphane can reverse this decline. This means broccoli may keep your immune system in tiptop shape, allowing it to stave off viruses and cancer.

Targets cancer cells. Researchers from the Linus Pauling Institute at Oregon State University discovered that sulforaphane operates like an elite Special Forces unit, selectively targeting and killing cancer cells while leaving normal prostate cells alone. It works by inhibiting histone deacetylase (HDAC) enzymes. These enzymes can affect DNA and stifle certain genes, including tumor suppressor genes. This allows runaway cell growth, a feature of cancer. But HDAC inhibitors — like sulforaphane — can help trigger these genes and restore order.

To fight cancer, make room for broccoli in your diet. Aim for three to five servings a week. But don't stop there. You can give broccoli an extra boost when you pair it with something spicy, like mustard, horseradish, or wasabi. That's because these foods contain myrosinase, an enzyme needed in order to form sulforaphane.

A University of Illinois study found that combining broccoli powder with fresh broccoli sprouts enhanced absorption of sulforaphane. Broccoli powder does not contain sulforaphane but does contain its precursor, glucoraphanin. Broccoli sprouts, on the other hand, are chock-full of myrosinase. The combination resulted in much higher levels of sulforaphane than either one would yield on its own. Other foods that contain myrosinase include radishes, arugula, cabbage, watercress, and Brussels sprouts.

How you prepare broccoli also matters. When you overcook it, you destroy the myrosinase. Steaming broccoli for two to four minutes will preserve the enzyme and other nutrients.

Brew a cup of prostate protection

Your morning coffee ritual might just save your life. A solid study links coffee, both regular and decaf, to a much lower risk of lethal prostate cancer.

The Health Professionals Follow-Up Study makes a compelling argument for indulging in coffee. More than 47,000 men were studied for 20 years. In the end, those who drank the most coffee — 6 or more cups a day — were:

- nearly 20 percent less likely to get prostate cancer at all.
- half as likely to end up with advanced prostate cancer.
- a whopping 60 percent less likely to develop a deadly form of prostate cancer.

Coffee may not prevent prostate cancer completely, but it may ward off the most deadly and aggressive forms of the disease. This eye-opening beverage can cause big changes in your body — all for the better.

Balances blood sugar. Coffee is packed with compounds called chlorogenic acids that inhibit glucose absorption in the intestines. They may also fiddle with hormones in your gut that affect how your cells respond to insulin. Plus, coffee contains lignans, powerful antioxidants that improve blood sugar management.

Balancing your blood sugar matters, because excess insulin encourages the growth of cancer cells. Men who have too much insulin in their bloodstream are much more likely to see their prostate cancer progress, or to die from it.

Boosts testosterone. Drinking coffee may raise your testosterone levels. More testosterone can be bad early on. This hormone may feed prostate cancer growth in the beginning, but some experts think it may help keep the disease from getting worse later on.

A cup of Joe also seems to increase the amount of sex hormone-binding globulin (SHBG) in the body. Data from 18 studies links high SHBG with a lower risk of prostate cancer.

Squashes inflammation. Coffee is a top source of antioxidants that crushed inflammation in a study. Scientists think inflammation has a big hand in the development of prostate cancer. It can cause early-stage cancerous lesions to pop up in the prostate. Coffee antioxidants can quiet inflammation and lower the risk of advanced prostate cancer.

Of course, one study doesn't make an airtight case. But researchers have analyzed other data on coffee that suggests it reduces the likelihood of developing the disease. Still, more studies are needed to confirm their results. So if you enjoy coffee, there's little harm and potentially a lot of help in each cup.

Even a small amount of coffee is beneficial. Drinking 1 to 3 cups a day slashed men's risk of advanced cancer by 25 percent and lethal cancer by almost 30 percent.

Tasty juice puts the squeeze on disease

Pomegranates may have a unique power to slow the progression of prostate cancer. And drinking the juice of this fruit, which is easily found online or in your local supermarket, may be one of the best ways to get this benefit.

This juice is a top source of antioxidants, including flavonoids and tannins. In fact, its antioxidants are much more powerful than the ones in red wine, and about as potent as those in green tea. In lab studies, extracts made from pomegranate blocked the growth of prostate, colon, breast, and lung cancer cells. In particular, pomegranate:

- triggered cancer cells to literally self-destruct, a process called apoptosis.
- blocked prostate cancer cells from multiplying like crazy.
- kept these cells from metastasizing, or spreading to other areas.
- increased the chance of surviving prostate cancer, at least in animal studies.

Because the fruit packs so many healthful compounds — phenols, flavonoids, anthocyanins, and tannins, to name a few — experts aren't sure which ones get the credit. Most likely they work together, squashing cancer in different ways.

Buying a supplement that boasts only one of these compounds probably won't give you the same protection as eating the whole fruit. The juice, however, might.

In one study, researchers fed two groups of mice pomegranate juice in their water. The mice, who were genetically engineered to develop prostate cancer, got the human equivalent of 8.5 to 17 ounces (about one to two glasses) of juice each day. A third group drank only plain water. Not surprisingly, all of the mice in the water-only group ended up with prostate cancer. Only half of the mice getting "two glasses" of pomegranate juice daily developed the disease. Their cancer was also much less likely to metastasize and spread.

This fruit may not prevent prostate cancer altogether, but it could save a life simply by delaying the disease. That alone may be reason enough for nearly every man to start drinking it. Prostate cancer most often strikes older men, and it's generally slow-growing. Slowing it down even further could allow many men to reach the natural end of their lives before the cancer becomes a serious problem.

Did you know?

Pomegranates aren't the only fruit that could be good for your prostate. Cranberries, long known for fighting urinary tract infections, may also battle cancer. More research is needed, but cranberries have crushed prostate cancer cells in lab studies. Look for products that are made from the whole berries. These contain the most cancer-fighting compounds.

Safer ways to eat red meat

Grilling your meat until it's well done could give you aggressive prostate cancer. Scientists polled nearly 1,000 men, asking them how often they ate meat and how they cooked it.

Those who ate the most red meat were more likely to develop aggressive prostate cancer. In fact, eating the most ground beef or processed meat seemed to double a man's risk. What mattered most, however, was not the meat itself but how it had been cooked.

Blame open flames. Eating beef, hamburger, or chicken cooked over an open flame worsened the men's chances of aggressive prostate cancer. The more they ate, the greater the danger.

- Men who ate the most barbecued beef were 60 percent more likely to develop this disease compared with men who ate no flame-grilled meat.
- Those who ate the most barbecued hamburgers were 86 percent more likely to get prostate cancer.
- Ground meat that had not been grilled or barbecued, however, had almost no impact on risk.

Smoking and grilling over an open flame forms cancer-causing compounds called polycyclic aromatic hydrocarbons (PAHs). As meat cooks, the fat and juices drip down into the flames. Drippings cause the flames to flare up and lick the meat — flames that contain PAHs. Enzymes in your body then turn the PAHs coating your meat into cancerous compounds.

Avoid overcooking at high temps. Flames aren't all, though. Researchers also compared men who took their grilled meat rare or medium with those who ate their meat well-done and very well-done.

Men who liked their red meat with some pink in it were no more likely to get aggressive prostate cancer than men who never ate grilled meat. Men who ate a lot of well-done and very well-done red meat, on the other hand, were more than twice as likely to develop this disease.

The danger comes from heating meat to a high temperature or cooking it for a long time. Under these conditions, the creatine, proteins, and sugars in meat react to form heterocyclic amines (HCAs), potentially cancerous compounds.

Of course, undercooked meat poses its own threats. So instead of eating it rare, try these surefire ways to reduce HCAs.

- Preheat meat. Precooking meat in the microwave for just one minute will remove most of the compounds that cause HCAs.
- Flip frequently. Turn your meat on the grill more often, to keep the cooking temperature lower.
- Remember to marinate. Research shows that marinades containing red wine, garlic, onions, or lemon juice dramatically cut down on the formation of cancer-causing compounds.

Lemony herb meat marinade

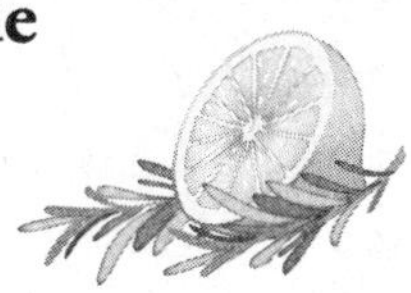

1/4 cup olive oil

1/4 cup fresh lemon juice

1 teaspoon lemon zest

1 large onion, chopped

3 cloves garlic, finely chopped

2 tablespoons fresh rosemary, chopped;
or 1 tablespoon dried rosemary

3/4 teaspoon freshly ground pepper

Mix all the ingredients in a bowl and pour them into a sealable plastic bag. Place the meat in the bag, and turn to coat. Refrigerate for two to eight hours, turning occasionally. When ready to grill, throw out the used marinade. Do not reuse it for basting.

One bright spice outsmarts cancer

Turmeric is a delicious spice used to flavor curries, soups, and stews. Commonly used in Indian and Southeast Asian cuisine, it gets its dazzling yellow color from curcumin — a compound that brings a slew of health benefits. In fact, test tube and animal research suggest curcumin may even aid in prostate cancer prevention. One study showed that curcumin:

- kept prostate cancer cells from multiplying.
- prevented them from spreading, or metastasizing, to other areas.
- blocked inflammation, stopping cancer from developing in the first place and triggering existing cancer cells to self-destruct.

These potent effects have experts excited that curcumin could help prevent, and one day even treat, prostate cancer. Scientists say this compound could work alongside traditional cancer treatments, such as radiation.

Unfortunately, your body doesn't absorb curcumin very well. You have to eat a lot of it for even a small amount to reach your bloodstream. However, punching up your favorite turmeric-infused meal with other seasonings can help you absorb more.

Adding black pepper to your curry, for instance, can boost your body's absorption of curcumin by a whopping 2,000 percent. Other seasonings, including fresh dill weed, dried oregano, fresh cilantro, and red onions are top sources of quercetin, another compound that brings in more curcumin.

Turmeric is no slacker when it comes to other cancers, either. Check out the "Did you know?" box in the *Breast cancer* chapter to see how curcumin battles other cancers.

> Adding flaxseeds to your morning oatmeal could help kill cancer cells dead in their tracks. Research suggests that these tiny seeds may prevent prostate cancer tumors from growing.

Respiratory disease

Live longer with these hearty favorites

Fiber-rich foods may have more power than you ever imagined. A study of more than 300,000 people ages 50 to 71 found that those who ate more fiber were less likely to die from heart disease, infectious diseases, and respiratory diseases like chronic obstructive pulmonary disease (COPD).

In fact, men who ate the most fiber had a 31 percent lower risk of death from a respiratory disease than men who ate the least fiber. For women who ate the most fiber, that risk was 46 percent lower.

Fiber may help because it has surprising anti-inflammatory powers. Scientists have found that people who eat a lot of fiber have lower levels of inflammatory markers in their systems. That's important because inflammation may cause COPD to become worse over time. That may be one reason why the fiber lovers in the study were less likely to die from COPD.

> Don't add a lot of fiber all at once. That leads to uncomfortable side effects like gas, diarrhea, cramps, and bloating. Add fiber to your diet gradually, and drink plenty of water.

You can add fiber to your diet by eating more fruits, nuts, seeds, and vegetables. Fiber from grains may be particularly helpful, the researchers report. If you often eat low-fiber foods, changes like these may help you.

- Switch from Cream of Wheat, Rice Krispies, or another low-fiber cereal to oatmeal from rolled oats or steel-cut oats.

Or enjoy a hot cereal of cooked brown rice with cinnamon and raisins.

- Try barley as a side dish, a hot breakfast cereal, or add it to soups, stews, or casseroles. To cook 1 cup of pearled barley, boil 3 cups of water, add the barley, and bring to a boil again. Cover and cook on low for 45 minutes or until tender.
- Add 1/2 cup of uncooked oatmeal to each pound of ground beef you use to form hamburgers.
- Check the fiber grams and serving size on your pasta package. Next time you shop, look for pasta with more fiber. Do the same for your sandwich bread, rolls, and waffles.
- Try less familiar, high-fiber grains, such as bulgur and spelt.
- Eat brown rice instead of white rice.

Think zinc to ward off pneumonia

More than a million people in the United States are hospitalized with pneumonia every year, but you don't have to be one of them. A study by Boston scientists reveals that a smart way to avoid pneumonia is to "think zinc."

Earlier research showed that older adults are often deficient in zinc, and that low zinc levels may contribute to age-related problems with the immune system. When your immune system is impaired, you have a harder time fighting off diseases like pneumonia.

The Boston researchers found this to be true. Nursing home residents who had low blood levels of zinc at the end of a yearlong study had a higher risk of pneumonia than residents with normal levels. Their pneumonia also lasted longer. Although all the participants took a daily multivitamin containing 7 milligrams (mg) of zinc, only those whose zinc levels rose to normal lowered their chances of pneumonia by the end of the study.

To increase your zinc supply and help shield yourself from pneumonia, try these simple but mighty foods.

Food	Amount	Milligrams of zinc
cooked wild oysters	6 medium	51.9
Total whole-grain cereal	1 cup	17.5
canned baked beans with pork and tomato sauce	1 cup	13.9
trail mix with chocolate chips, salted nuts, and seeds	1 cup	7.1
braised beef chuck pot roast	3 ounces	6.6
Alaska king crab	3 ounces	6.5
braised lamb shoulder roast	3 ounces	6.2
broiled lean ground beef	3 ounces	5.5
canned blue crab	1 cup	5.1
braised pork spare ribs	3 ounces	3.9

The researchers caution that the extra 7 mg a day of zinc only brought some of the study participants back to normal levels. If you feel like you're not getting enough from foods, ask your doctor if you can safely take zinc supplements. Just be aware that these supplements, when taken over a long period and in high doses, can lead to a copper deficiency.

HEALTH ALERT!

Beans and whole grains may be marvelously nutritious foods, but they are not your best sources of zinc. Both contain the substance phytic acid, which may keep your body from absorbing up to 50 percent of the zinc in foods. This doesn't mean you shouldn't eat beans and whole grains. In fact, you should eat whole grains every day. Just don't use beans or whole grains as your main source of zinc.

Surprising relief for asthma attacks

You're halfway through the plane flight when your asthma starts acting up, and you suddenly realize you forgot to pack your inhaler. Don't panic. Ask for a cup of hot coffee, instead.

The caffeine in coffee is a mild bronchodilator, meaning it can help open up your airways. In fact, a review of research concluded that caffeine can modestly improve lung function if you have mild-to-moderate asthma. Caffeine temporarily raises measures of lung function for up to four hours.

This solution works best if you drink at least 5 milligrams (mg) of caffeine for every 2.2 pounds of your body weight. That would be roughly 250 mg, or about 2 cups, for a 110-pound woman. Hot coffee is a good source of this caffeine because cold beverages can help trigger an asthma attack.

Using a rescue asthma inhaler is far more effective than coffee if you have an asthma attack. But when an inhaler is not available, a cup or two of caffeinated coffee at the start of an attack may help you breathe better and possibly save your life.

Did you know?

It's 5 p.m. somewhere — time for the daily commute. Ever think what rush-hour pollution might be doing to your airways? If you have asthma, contaminated particles seeping into your car's ventilation system can trigger inflammation and worsen your symptoms.

Now consider this. It may sound unbelievable, but it's true. You can keep your asthma at bay by loading up on broccoli. According to one study, the sulforaphane provided in about a cup of cooked broccoli can boost your cells' antioxidant ability and your anti-inflammatory response to air pollutants. And the quercetin in this vegetable puts the brakes on your body's histamine production and blocks inflammation.

Simple way to keep aging lungs strong

Fish may be famous as heart food, and milk may be good for your bones, but now scientists think these foods may have a nutrient that can help your lungs, too — vitamin D.

Improves lung function. New Zealand researchers studied the information collected on more than 14,000 participants in the U.S. National Health and Nutrition Examination Survey (NHANES). The researchers discovered that people with the highest blood levels of vitamin D had significantly better lung function than people with the lowest levels. In fact, vitamin D made a bigger difference in lung function than not smoking did.

Fights harmful changes. Some experts have suggested vitamin D may help fight against lung tissue remodeling, the damaging changes to your lungs caused by pollution, cigarette smoke, or other irritants. That would be good news if they're right because lung tissue remodeling eventually leads to breathing problems and chronic obstructive pulmonary disease (COPD).

Strengthens breathing muscles. Another study suggests vitamin D may strengthen your breathing muscles. Belgian researchers recruited 50 people with COPD whose symptoms had been getting worse. Although all participants enrolled in a three-month pulmonary rehabilitation program, only half took a monthly vitamin D supplement while the rest took a placebo. The supplement was equal to roughly 3,300 international units of vitamin D daily. By the end of the study, those taking vitamin D supplements showed significantly more improvement in the strength of their breathing muscles and capacity to exercise.

More research is needed to find out whether vitamin D can truly help fight breathing problems like COPD. In the meantime, try eating these tasty, vitamin-D-rich foods to see what this nutrient can do for you.

- 3 ounces of rainbow trout or smoked Chinook salmon
- chocolate milk or reduced-fat milk with added vitamin D
- canned pink salmon or canned light tuna
- filet of Atlantic or Pacific halibut
- canned clam chowder or tomato soup prepared with milk
- vitamin-D-fortified cereals such as Total Whole Grain or Kellogg's All-Bran

Since it's still too early to tell whether vitamin D from foods is enough to make a difference to your lungs, ask your doctor if you could benefit from vitamin D supplements as well.

Natural way to protect your lungs

Add some new fruits to your diet. Some studies have linked eating more fruits and vegetables with a drop in lung-related symptoms and lung disease. These studies even suggest certain compounds in fruit may help reduce allergy-caused asthma.

To put this to the test, New Zealand researchers pitted several black currant extracts against compounds that contribute to lung inflammation and asthma symptoms. In their test tube studies, black currant extract rich in antioxidants called proanthocyanidins suppressed a key substance that causes lungs to swell up. This means black currant compounds have the potential to help lessen the inflammation in your airways that can trigger asthma.

By learning how these plant chemicals affect the cells in your lungs, scientists might also be able to develop functional foods that could reduce the risk of asthma or allergies.

This research is in its early stages but has exciting possibilities for the future. Stay tuned.

Restless legs syndrome

Natural solutions for restless legs

It's hard to believe clams and chili are powerful enough to help quiet your restless legs, but scientists say the food you eat can have a big impact on how well you sleep.

Experts suspect a shortage of the brain chemical dopamine causes the symptoms of restless legs syndrome (RLS). But your body must have iron to produce dopamine. So if you don't get enough iron in your diet, you may not make enough dopamine either. In fact, up to 75 percent of people with RLS symptoms have low iron levels.

Not everyone who has RLS is iron deficient. That means increasing iron intake may not help unless you are already short on iron, so talk to your doctor about testing your iron levels. If you have a very severe deficiency, you may need iron supplements. But if your iron deficiency is less severe, experts recommend you try to get more iron from food before you try a supplement.

To mine the most iron from food, use these tips:

- Know the facts. Iron comes in two versions — heme iron and nonheme iron. Your body can draw more iron from foods with heme iron. You'll find high levels of this nutrient in clams, oysters, organ meats, beef, fish, pork, and poultry. One easy way to sneak more iron into your diet is to add canned clams to your spaghetti sauce while it cooks.
- Pair them up. To absorb more iron from foods that only

have nonheme iron, pair them with heme iron foods. For example, kidney beans only have nonheme iron, but you absorb more iron from them if they are cooked and eaten as part of beef chili. Other nonheme foods include pasta, dark green leafy vegetables like spinach and kale, dried peas and beans, seeds, nuts, and dried fruits.

- Boost absorption. Just 6 ounces of orange juice can double the amount of iron your body absorbs from nonheme iron foods. That means orange juice may help you calm your twitchy legs and get more sweet slumber. Drink orange juice with your cereal and milk, or eggs and toast. The vitamin C from the juice helps your body absorb nonheme iron from iron fortified-cereals, dairy products, breads, and eggs. Other good sources of vitamin C include cranberry juice, strawberries, sweet peppers, broccoli, oranges, kiwifruit, tomatoes, and tomato paste.

Did you know?

Do your legs have varicose veins? If so, you'll want to listen up. The cramps and throbbing associated with this condition may prevent you from getting a good night's sleep — just like restless legs syndrome could. In fact, some research suggests a connection between these two conditions.

That's where extracts of a shrub called Butcher's broom come in. This natural remedy may be the easiest way to sweep away the pain and swelling of varicose veins. It can strengthen and firm veins, too. Just be sure to talk with your doctor before taking this product.

Rheumatoid arthritis

Snack on cherries to soothe aches

Like an ice cream sundae, the list of foods that fight arthritis has a cherry on top. This fruit isn't only delicious, it's medicinal too. That's because this little-known home remedy is loaded with compounds that help you eat away your pain.

Besides great taste, cherries have plenty of scientific support. Credit goes to anthocyanins, the antioxidant pigments that give cherries their red color. These powerful flavonoids block enzymes in the body that cause inflammation and pain.

Studies suggest that cherries can be a safe and tasty alternative to nonsteroidal anti-inflammatory drugs (NSAIDS), common remedies for arthritis pain. They may also help with other inflammatory conditions, including gout and muscle pain. Here's a quick rundown of the cheery news about cherries.

- Researchers at Michigan State University found that the anthocyanins in cherries stopped inflammation just as well as ibuprofen and naproxen — but without the unpleasant side effects. In fact, at certain concentrations, tart cherry juice is 10 times more effective than aspirin in treating arthritis pain and inflammation.
- Scientists at the Agricultural Research Service (ARS) shed more light on how cherries work. In one small study, 18 healthy people who ate about 45 fresh Bing cherries a day for a month had significant reductions in blood levels of C-reactive protein, nitric oxide, and a marker for T-cell activation called RANTES — all indicators of inflammation.

Interestingly, cherries seem to selectively target some inflammatory compounds while not affecting others.

- In a previous study of 10 women, ARS researchers found that eating 45 Bing cherries in one sitting lowered blood levels of urate, a precursor of the painful uric acid crystals that accumulate in the joints of people with gout. The cherries also brought down levels of C-reactive protein and nitric oxide.
- Other studies reported that drinking tart cherry juice minimizes muscle pain and reduces the symptoms of muscle damage during exercise.

As you can see, cherries pack a lot of power into a small package. Eating fresh cherries or drinking cherry juice can help squelch inflammation, soothe arthritis pain, and sidestep gout and muscle damage. Make room in your eating plan for more cherries, and you'll give your joints a treat.

12 foods that fight pain

While cherries have been the most studied food, they're not the only source of anthocyanins. To boost your anthocyanin intake and soothe arthritis symptoms, try these delicious foods.

- blackberries
- blueberries
- red grapes
- red raspberries
- strawberries
- cranberries
- plums
- black currants
- red cabbage
- red onions
- blood orange juice
- purple sweet potatoes

Remarkable ways to fight RA

Safecracking can land you in prison — but walnuts represent a form of "safe cracking" that can help you escape from the prison of rheumatoid arthritis (RA). But don't stop there. Add olive oil and fish to your meal plan, too. Here's why.

Go nuts. When you crack open a walnut, you help take a crack against inflammation, a key component of RA. What's the secret to walnuts' success? Unlike other nuts, they contain a ton of omega-3 fatty acids. Specifically, they contain alpha-linolenic acid, the plant form of omega-3s. An ounce of walnuts gives you about 2.5 grams of omega-3s.

Adding walnuts and flaxseed oil, another source of alpha-linolenic acid, to your diet can reduce your levels of C-reactive protein, a marker of inflammation linked to arthritis and heart disease. As a bonus, the omega-3s in walnuts also help lower your blood pressure. That's important because people with RA have a higher risk of heart disease.

Opt for olive oil. Another surprising source of omega-3s is olive oil. You may already know that olive oil boasts plenty of heart-healthy monounsaturated fat, but it also contains small amounts of alpha-linolenic acid, about 0.1 gram per tablespoon. Yet, this tiny amount can make a big difference.

Research shows that olive oil limits the production of harmful free radicals and neutralizes those that are produced during inflammation. Swap olive oil for other vegetable oils, and you'll help restore the balance between pro-inflammatory omega-6 fatty acids and anti-inflammatory omega-3s. This simple step should help ward off a host of conditions marked by chronic inflammation, including RA.

Feast on fish. Sorry, landlubbers, but the best source of omega-3 fatty acids remains fish. For the most omega-3s, choose fatty fish like salmon, tuna, herring, and mackerel. Anchovies, bluefish, carp, catfish, halibut, lake trout, sea bass, and whitefish are also good choices.

Fish oil supplements should also do the trick. Several studies showed that fish oil supplements can improve morning stiffness and joint tenderness in people with rheumatoid arthritis. For even better results, some researchers suggest combining fish oil with nonsteroidal anti-inflammatory drugs (NSAIDs), like aspirin or ibuprofen. However, these studies have not lasted beyond three months. Well designed, long-term studies are needed to confirm these results.

> One in 28 women and one in 59 men will develop rheumatoid arthritis during their lifetimes, according to the Mayo Clinic. Risk is highest for people between ages 60 and 80.

In the meantime, make sure to fit more omega-3 fatty acids into your diet. Whether you get your omega-3s from fish, fish oil supplements, or plant sources like walnuts or olive oil, you'll be doing your joints a favor.

4 things you should know before eating fish

All the super nutritious omega-3 fatty acids in fish are important because they help fight inflammation and guard against a variety of health problems, including arthritis. Unfortunately, though, eating fish can leave you a little green around the gills.

That's because fish may contain high levels of mercury or toxic chemicals called polychlorinated biphenyls (PCBs). Here's what you need to know about these risks — and how to sidestep them.

Go wild or stay on the farm? Where you get your fish could make a difference. In general, wild-caught fish — especially larger fish that eat smaller fish — may have higher levels of mercury, while farmed fish come with much higher levels of PCBs.

There are other factors to consider. Wild fish have higher levels of omega-3s, but they also cost more and may not be available at all times. Farmed fish are cheaper and widely available but higher in pro-inflammatory omega-6 fatty acids. That's due to their feed, which may contain corn or soy.

Ultimately, it's up to you whether to eat wild or farmed fish. Both come with plenty of benefits and a few drawbacks.

Did you know?

Don't eat foods high in purines if you have gout. Found in certain meats, fish, and other foods, purines are broken down into uric acid by your body. Deposits of uric acid crystals can build up in your joints, usually your big toe, and cause serious pain.

One way to limit purines is to swap meat for a protein-rich, vegetable-based meat substitute. But a Czech study discovered that not all of these products are created equal. The type of protein makes a big difference. Purine levels are higher in mycoprotein or soybean-based products, but lower in wheat protein or egg white-based products. Make sure to read labels carefully.

You should also avoid purine-rich foods like anchovies, asparagus, cauliflower, dried beans and peas, gravy, herring, liver, mackerel, mushrooms, poultry, sardines, scallops, and spinach. Limit alcohol intake, but drink plenty of other fluids — including milk — to help flush out the uric acid.

Minimize mercury. This heavy metal, which is especially harmful to unborn or young children, is found in virtually all fish. But some fish contain higher levels than others. That's why the U.S. Food and Drug Administration has warned pregnant or nursing women to avoid eating high-mercury fish. Shark, king mackerel, tilefish, ahi tuna, and swordfish fall into this category.

Change it up. Variety is the spice of life — and a good strategy when it comes to eating seafood. Eat a variety of fish to reduce your risk of exposure to any one contaminant. Safer, low-mercury choices include shrimp, anchovies, catfish, clams, cod, crabs, flounder, haddock, pollock, salmon, sardines, scallops, and canned light tuna.

HEALTH ALERT!

A bucket of popcorn at the theater may sound like a good idea at the time, but you may regret that salty snack after the movie is over.

That's because some studies suggest salt may prompt several autoimmune diseases, including rheumatoid arthritis, psoriasis, multiple sclerosis, and ankylosing spondylitis, or arthritis of the spine.

Yale School of Medicine researchers discovered the link between a high-salt diet and autoimmune conditions when they conducted an animal study. They say too much salt caused the animals to produce inflammatory cells closely associated with autoimmune diseases. These cells attack healthy tissue.

To keep your sodium intake down, cook from scratch so you can control just how much salt is in your food. Swap out some of the salt in recipes and get flavor from herbs, spices, or a squeeze of citrus juice. If you're buying prepackaged food, look for low-sodium options.

Trim the fat. How you prepare your fish also makes a difference. Removing the skin and visible fat will help get rid of some PCBs. Grill, broil, or bake your fish so the fat can drip away while it cooks.

Remember, the health benefits of fish far outweigh any potential dangers. So don't avoid this food. You should still aim for at least two fish meals a week. Just take some precautions to tip the scales even further in the right direction.

'D'-fend yourself from arthritis

A bowl of cereal in the morning can help fortify you for the day ahead. As long as the cereal and milk have been fortified with vitamin D, your breakfast may also fortify your immune system against rheumatoid arthritis (RA).

Vitamin D may help your body resist rheumatoid arthritis by fighting inflammation and regulating your immune system so it doesn't spiral out of control and attack your body.

Realize the risk. Low levels of vitamin D have been linked to rheumatoid arthritis and other autoimmune diseases, including multiple sclerosis and Crohn's disease. Both geography and diet could contribute to a vitamin D deficiency.

- A Boston University study found that women living in the northeastern United States — places like New Hampshire, Vermont, and Maine — were more likely to develop RA than those in sunnier climates. The difference may be a lack of vitamin D, which your body makes from sunlight.
- Previously, a study of nearly 30,000 women suggested that women whose diets included more vitamin D had a lower risk of developing RA. Women who got less than 200 international units (IU) of vitamin D each day had a 33 percent greater risk of developing the disease.

Increase your intake. Spending more time in the sun is the easiest way to boost your vitamin D levels. You can also take vitamin D supplements. Look for vitamin D3, the form naturally produced by your skin.

But the tastiest way to get more vitamin D is through your diet. Good food sources include fatty fish like salmon, herring, mackerel, sardines, and tuna. Fortified foods, such as milk, cheese, orange juice, and cereal, also provide vitamin D. You can even get a small amount from mushrooms and egg yolks.

Sunshine, supplements, and super food sources can all up your vitamin D intake — and that's a good strategy to keep RA down.

Blood test spots RA early

Early diagnosis and treatment gives you an edge against rheumatoid arthritis (RA). But identifying RA early can be quite difficult because the symptoms resemble those of several other conditions.

Luckily, your doctor can order a simple blood test if he suspects that you might have RA. This type of testing looks for abnormal types and levels of antibodies in the blood — warning signs of the disease.

Sarcopenia

Protect your muscles with protein

With age comes wisdom — and, unfortunately, muscle loss. Prevent this problem by getting plenty of protein. Your muscles, bones, hair, and skin all need this essential nutrient. Find out how much you need and which foods you should eat.

Stop sarcopenia. Sarcopenia refers to the gradual, age-related loss of muscle and strength. Older people lose about 3 percent of their lean body mass every 10 years, leaving them weaker and more susceptible to falls, fractures, and other dangers. Sarcopenia also makes it harder to perform everyday tasks, like carrying groceries or just getting around. Experts estimate that as many as 50 percent of people age 80 and older have sarcopenia.

Push back with protein. Put more protein on your plate, and you'll maintain more of your strength. Your body needs protein to build muscle and bone, and you might need even more as you get older to combat sarcopenia and osteoporosis.

One study found that seniors who ate more protein were less likely to suffer hip fractures. Those who got the least amount of protein in their diet had approximately 50 percent more hip fractures than those who got enough. That's likely because protein helps build stronger muscles in your legs, which could help reduce the risk of falls.

The key is not only to boost your overall protein intake but to make sure you eat protein throughout the day — starting with breakfast. You should get at least .36 grams of protein for every pound you weigh. Ideally, you want about 15 to 30 grams of protein with each meal. A 3-ounce serving of beef, turkey breast, or salmon will go a long way in helping you to reach that goal.

Pick from plenty of sources. You can get protein from both animal and plant sources. For animal sources, choose lean meat, poultry, fish, milk, yogurt, cheese, and eggs. Good plant sources include nuts, seeds, legumes, grains, and tofu. If you have trouble chewing or digesting meat, these softer vegetable sources could come in handy.

Talk to your doctor before drastically boosting your protein intake. If you have kidney disease, for instance, a high-protein diet may be dangerous.

Did you know?

You can guard against sarcopenia by building up the muscles you already have. Weight lifting, or resistance exercise, can help keep you strong and steady as you age.

One study found that six months of resistance exercise can reverse signs of aging in the skeletal muscles of older people. Besides making you stronger, resistance training also preserves your independence, since it improves your ability to climb stairs or get up out of a chair. It can also improve coordination, which can help you avoid falls.

For best results, combine your strength training with stretching. And take it slow. Austrian researchers found that "super-slow" resistance exercise works even better to maintain muscle mass and strength.

You don't even need barbells to improve your strength and balance. A Chinese study found that tai chi improved muscle strength around the ankles and knees.

Secret to sidestepping falls

Stay on your feet with a cold, refreshing treat. Simply pour yourself a glass of milk — a tasty drink that can cut your risk of falling nearly in half. Just make sure your milk is fortified with vitamin D.

Decrease falls with D. Several studies show that vitamin D has a positive effect on muscle strength and balance. A Swiss study of 378 people aged 65 and older found that those who received a daily vitamin D supplement — and also got enough calcium — were 55 percent less likely to fall than those who took a placebo. Of course, milk provides both calcium and vitamin D, so you get a double dose of protection.

More recently, an analysis of eight previous studies determined that vitamin D supplements could reduce the risk of falls by up to 26 percent. Aim for between 600 and 800 international units (IU) of vitamin D a day. Keep in mind that vitamin D3 may be more effective than vitamin D2. As always, talk to your doctor before taking any dietary supplements.

Make muscles stronger. Muscle weakness is a risk factor for falls and also a symptom of vitamin D deficiency. That could help explain why boosting vitamin D intake can also boost your strength and keep you upright.

An Australian study shed more light on how vitamin D helps. The yearlong study included 302 women aged 70 to 90 who had low blood levels of vitamin D. They received either 1,000 IU of vitamin D2 or a placebo each day. Both groups also received 1,000 milligrams of calcium a day.

Researchers found that vitamin D supplements helped improve hip muscle strength and mobility in those who were the slowest and weakest at the start of the study. Mobility was measured by the Timed Up and Go Test (TUAG), which involves getting up from a chair, walking three meters (about 10 feet), turning around, returning to the chair, and sitting down again.

Select several sources. Milk and supplements aren't the only ways to get vitamin D. Spending five to 30 minutes in the sun a few times a week can help boost your vitamin D levels. You can also get vitamin D from liver, egg yolks, and oily fish like salmon, mackerel, tuna, and sardines. Besides milk, foods fortified with vitamin D include orange juice and breakfast cereals.

Simple way to fight sarcopenia

Looking for an easy way to save your muscles? Go fish. A promising study suggests that omega-3 fatty acids — those are the kind found in fish — may help prevent or treat sarcopenia by stimulating muscle protein synthesis in older people.

In the study, 16 people age 65 or over received either a high-dose omega-3 fatty acid supplement or a corn oil placebo daily for eight weeks. The omega-3 supplement, called Lovaza, is available by prescription and provides 4 grams of the fatty acids found in fish oil. Although researchers aren't sure exactly how omega-3s work, these fatty acids may boost muscle by increasing the activation of a key signaling pathway involved in muscle cell growth.

More research is needed, but adding more fish oil to your diet could be a simple, safe way to counteract muscle loss. Besides supplements, you can get omega-3s from fatty fish like salmon, mackerel, herring, and tuna.

Shingles

Cut your odds with fruits and veggies

Add pineapple slices to a ham sandwich, cranberry sauce to a turkey sandwich, or sautéed peppers, onions, and carrots to your spaghetti sauce. These changes will add more flavor to your food. Not only that — they may help you avoid shingles.

A British study found that people who ate less than one piece of fruit a week were three times more likely to develop shingles than those who ate more than three servings of fruit a day. And for people over age 60, the fewer vegetables they ate, the higher their risk of getting this painful condition.

Shingles risk also rises for those over 60 who got lower amounts of vitamin A, vitamin B6, vitamin C, vitamin E, folic acid, iron, and zinc. The researchers suggest that age weakens your immune system and its resistance to the shingles virus.

You probably faced this virus before if you had chicken pox. Your immune system conquered the symptoms within a few weeks but could not get rid of the virus. So this *herpes varicella-zoster* virus stayed in your body, waiting for your immune system to become weak enough to defeat. Sometimes, that never happens. But if age or other issues weaken your immune system enough, the virus triggers shingles.

The British researchers suspect fruits, vegetables, and the vitamins and minerals they contain help defend your immune system against age-related weakening, making you less vulnerable to shingles.

But this only works if you eat enough fruits and vegetables. Start by making small changes like these.

- Add shredded peppers and carrots to chili.
- Slip thin apple slices into a peanut butter or ham sandwich.
- Add chopped vegetables to canned chicken noodle soup.

Try this sweet way to heal

Honey may be a fantastic natural way to help your shingles rash or blisters heal. It fights inflammation, helps stimulate your immune system, and may even boost your skin's ability to heal.

Remember, the shingles virus is essentially the recycled version of the chicken pox virus, *herpes varicella-zoster,* a member of the herpes virus family. One study showed that applying honey to sores caused by other herpes viruses healed those sores faster than the popular prescription treatment acyclovir. More research is needed to learn whether honey can have similar effects on shingles rashes. But a research review of therapies for shingles suggested honey may turn out to be a possible treatment.

The lack of scientific evidence hasn't stopped people from trying this unusual remedy. One woman says honey helped ease the burning and pain of shingles for up to eight hours. She applied raw, unfiltered honey to the affected areas, covered them with gauze, and placed a wrap over the gauze to protect her clothing and hold the gauze in place. When the pain returned, she removed the gauze and wrap, rinsed off the honey, and applied the treatment again.

Another supporter recommends spreading a light layer of honey over the shingles and letting it sit for at least an hour. After that, rinse with lukewarm water and gently blot the areas dry with a towel. He says you shouldn't use the heat-treated, nonorganic honey you find at the supermarket. Instead, buy raw, organic honey from a local beekeeper, at health food stores, or over the internet.

These homemade remedies may not be right for everyone, so talk to your doctor before you try one. But if she gives you the green light, you may find that honey means sweet relief.

HEALTH ALERT!

You're shopping for honey and its health benefits, but you end up with a container of high-fructose corn syrup. That's right — there are honey counterfeiters who dilute real honey with products like corn syrup to lower their production costs and outsell legitimate beekeepers with their cheaper products.

Although the U.S. Food and Drug Administration nabs some of this imported honey, some still makes it to store shelves. Testing honey for pollen content can reveal where the honey came from, but this testing is rare. Here's how to lower your odds of getting fake honey.

- Buy from a local beekeeper, farmer's market, co-op, or a natural foods store.
- Check for the name "Golden Heritage" on the back of the honey brand you buy. This honey distributor tests for pollen.
- Buy organic honey. In one test, most organic supermarket honey contained pollen.

Subdue shingles with the right foods

Remember the old saying, "feed a cold and starve a fever?" Some doctors and researchers think you can starve the shingles virus as well.

Cold sores and genital herpes are caused by *herpes simplex* viruses, cousins of the shingles virus *herpes varicella-zoster*. Several studies have shown that eating more of the amino acid lysine may help prevent cold sores and herpes outbreaks. This has led some experts to suggest lysine may also fight shingles.

The herpes virus needs another amino acid, arginine, to grow and multiply. But lysine constantly works to block arginine's effects, remove it from your body, and keep it out of your cells. This deprives the herpes virus of vital fuel — in other words, starving it.

So far, no studies have proven that lysine can defeat the shingles virus or help during an outbreak, but some people swear by it. One person says the reason he never needed pain medicine for shingles was because he immediately started taking antiviral medication, eating more lysine-rich foods, taking lysine supplements, and restricting arginine-rich foods. High-arginine foods include chocolate, nuts, oats, seeds, coconut, wheat, gelatin, and peanut butter.

Others say they avoided outbreaks or made them milder by limiting or excluding arginine-rich foods and eating more lysine-rich foods like yogurt. Other good sources of lysine are fish, vegetables, turkey, dairy, chicken, eggs, and beans.

Experts don't recommend you permanently remove arginine from your diet. But if you're prone to shingles outbreaks, try eating much more lysine than arginine. If it doesn't seem to help, ask your doctor if you can safely take lysine supplements. Some experts recommend 500 to 1,000 milligrams (mg) a day for prevention and 3,000 mg a day during outbreaks.

Sinusitis

Fend off pain with smart food choices

Sinus problems? Some foods can make you even more miserable, while others may help you feel better. Here's what you need to know.

Limit or avoid foods that hurt. Some foods help thicken mucus or cause swelling or dryness in your sinuses and nasal passages. That can help promote blocked sinuses, sinus pain, and even sinus infections. Be wary of these foods.

- Alcohol. You don't have to drink a lot of alcohol to trigger sinus problems. Even one or two drinks can harden your mucous membranes and cause swelling in your nasal passages and sinuses. Alcohol is also a diuretic that contributes to dehydration. That lack of liquid diminishes your body's ability to break down the mucus that blocks up your sinuses.
- Dairy products. Some experts think dairy products may thicken mucus or cause you to produce more than normal. Either one may prevent your sinuses from draining properly. Other experts find no evidence that dairy products affect mucus. But lactose intolerance, a sensitivity to the lactose in dairy products, may still cause sinus infections in some people. So try avoiding dairy products for a few weeks to see if you improve.
- Wheat and corn. As with milk, some experts think wheat and corn may contribute to thicker mucus or too much of it. Sinus problems can actually be one sign of an allergy to wheat or gluten. Try eliminating all foods with wheat and corn from your diet for a few weeks. If you start feeling better, you may have an intolerance or allergy to one of these foods.

Take advantage of foods that help. These foods and beverages may help your sinuses function properly and may undo some of the damage sinusitis causes.

- Water. Drink more water to help thin and loosen the hardened mucus blocking your sinuses so it can drain away properly. This also helps prevent congestion. Aim for at least six glasses a day.
- Chicken soup, hot tea, and other hot drinks. The steam from warm liquids can help break up congestion. What's more, ingredients in chicken soup have anti-inflammatory powers.

Guidelines restrict medicines

You may have to face your next sinus infection without antibiotics — and maybe even decongestants or antihistamines. The Infectious Diseases Society of America's (IDSA) treatment guidelines for sinusitis suggest that doctors only prescribe antibiotics if they see these signs of a bacterial sinus infection:

- Your symptoms have lasted 10 days or more, and you aren't getting better.
- You have severe symptoms such as a fever of at least 102 degrees Fahrenheit or a runny nose or face pain that has lasted three or four days.
- Your runny nose and other symptoms are getting worse, and you have new symptoms such as a fever and facial pain.

If your doctor prescribes antibiotics, the IDSA advises against using antihistamines or decongestants. Instead, your doctor should recommend drinking plenty of fluids, taking painkillers and fever fighters, rinsing your nose with saline solution, and taking a prescription nasal steroid to fight inflammation.

The "itis" part of sinusitis refers to inflammation, so a little anti-inflammatory chicken soup may be just what the doctor ordered.

- Onions, apples, and berries. These foods are sources of the flavonoid called quercetin. Quercetin has anti-inflammatory powers and can stabilize mast cells. So not only does it fight inflammation, it also blocks the release of histamines that cause allergy symptoms. To get more of this mighty nutrient in your diet, eat more blackberries, blueberries, onions, apples, broccoli, and kale. If you are not satisfied with the results after a few weeks, ask your doctor if you can safely take quercetin supplements.

Unstuff your stuffy nose naturally

Sinus problems were around long before Vicks VapoRub or minty "mentholated" nasal sprays. So why not try an old-fashioned version of these modern remedies? Solving your stuffy nose may be as simple as sipping a cup of peppermint tea.

Peppermint tea is made from the leaves of the peppermint plant, and those leaves contain a powerful compound called menthol. When you take a sip or a whiff of peppermint tea, those menthol vapors deliver their classic peppermint scent into your nose.

Once there, the menthol vapors interact with the cold receptors in your nose, making you feel as if more cool air is passing through your nostrils. This reduces that uncomfortable stuffed-up feeling and makes you feel as if you have taken a decongestant pill even though you haven't.

To take advantage of this effect, use this recipe the next time you have a stuffy nose.

- Measure out a tablespoon or two of fresh peppermint leaves or 2 to 3 teaspoons of dried peppermint leaves.

- Stir them into an 8-ounce cup of freshly boiled water.
- Let steep for 10 minutes.

Take a few sniffs of the rising steam while you wait. Add sweetener, if needed, and slowly sip the tea while it works its magic. You may be surprised at how much better you feel.

> **HEALTH ALERT!**
>
> If you have gastroesophageal reflux disease (GERD), drinking peppermint tea could make your symptoms worse. But you can still take advantage of peppermint's powers to help your clogged sinuses.
>
> Fill a bowl with steaming peppermint tea, or add a few drops of peppermint essential oil to a bowl of steaming hot water. Lean over the bowl, place a towel over your head, and breathe in the cool soothing scent. You can also try this with other herbs, like eucalyptus or thyme.

Sinus-soothing teas from your spice rack

You're out of peppermint tea but don't feel well enough to go out and buy more. Take advantage of some other options in your spice rack, instead.

Hot teas made from sage or fennel can help thin out the mucus that is stuffing up your sinuses. Even better, some compounds in fennel and anise may have anti-inflammatory powers, and sage is approved by Germany's Commission E as an active ingredient in gargles and mouthwashes for sore throats.

If you want fennel or anise tea, crush 1 teaspoon of fennel seeds or 1 1/2 teaspoons of anise seeds with a mortar and pestle. For sage tea, simply use 1 teaspoon of ground sage.

Bring 1 cup of water to a boil. Turn off the heat, and add your desired spice. Let steep for 10 to 15 minutes, then strain and drink.

Tasty tomato tonic

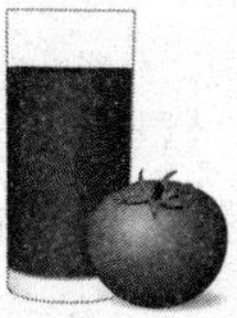

Some experts think a spiced warm drink like this one may help clear up sinus congestion.

1 cup (8 ounces) tomato juice

1 teaspoon chopped garlic

3/4 teaspoon lemon juice

1/4 teaspoon Tabasco sauce

Mix together, heat until very warm, and sip slowly.

Breathe easier with a common spice

Hot dog! Mustard eases many common respiratory problems. But it's not the bright yellow kind of mustard you squirt on frankfurters that helps you breathe better. Reach for dry, powdered mustard instead.

Cooking with this common spice can help ease chest congestion, bronchitis, bronchial cough, and sinusitis. Here are a few ways that mustard works its magic.

- Eating spicy foods — such as mustard, hot peppers, or horseradish — can clear your sinuses.
- Inhaling the steam from mustard also helps drain your clogged sinuses. Heat some onions and dry mustard in a little bit of oil. Fill a large bowl with hot water, then pour in the mustard mixture. Drape a towel over your head, close your eyes, and breathe deeply. Your nose should run, and you should cough up plenty of mucus.

- You don't even have to cook — or sniff — mustard to benefit from it. Mustard can also be used as a topical remedy for sinusitis and congestion.

You can make a paste from powdered mustard seeds, flour, and water. Wrap the mixture in linen, and lay it across your chest for 10 to 15 minutes to relieve congestion.

Mustard can irritate your skin, however, so think twice before trying this folk remedy. Rubbing olive oil on your skin after removing the paste may ease the irritation.

You can find dry mustard in the spice aisle of your supermarket. Use it to spice up your dishes — and to clear up your airways

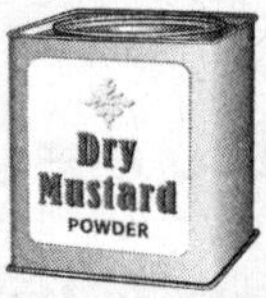

You bought dry mustard to help you through a sinus infection, but now you wonder what to do with the rest of the spice. Turn that dry mustard into regular mustard.

Combine three parts dry mustard with one part water and one part vinegar. Mix together, add a teaspoon of sugar or honey, and taste. Keep adding a little more sugar or honey until the mustard no longer tastes too hot. Store in a closed jar in the refrigerator.

When you have emptied that jar of nearly everything but the side scrapings, turn the remaining mustard into mustard vinaigrette salad dressing. Pour in 1/4 cup of vinegar, 3/4 cup of olive oil, and your favorite spices. Close the jar, shake to mix, and your mustard vinaigrette is ready.

Skin, hair & nail problems

Younger skin just a sweet potato away

You can tell the healthiest, most antioxidant-rich veggies and fruits by how they look and smell. There's no need to carry around a list of your best-bet foods. Simply pick the most brightly colored and strongly flavored fruits and vegetables. These are often the ones with the highest levels of phytochemicals, natural compounds in plants that can stimulate your immune system, prevent free radical damage, and protect you from cancer.

Make it orange — or red. Some of the best phytonutrients for skin protection are in the group called carotenoids, including beta carotene, lutein, and lycopene. You'll find carotenoids in abundance in red, orange, and green produce like carrots, sweet potatoes, tomatoes, winter squash, apricots, and broccoli.

High-carotenoid foods boost the antioxidant content of your skin to neutralize damaging free radicals from the sun's ultraviolet (UV) light, illness, drinking alcohol, and other stresses of everyday living. Studies show having more carotenoids in your skin can actually decrease the appearance of aging, such as skin furrows, wrinkles, and roughness.

Get a healthy glow. When you eat lots of high-carotenoid foods, it shows — all over your face. Experts found that people who eat more carotenoids have skin with a subtle golden glow, similar to the look of a slight tan. This was true in both light- and dark-skinned people. Researchers who studied how other people reacted to this skin coloring found they saw it as a healthy look, more attractive than a natural tan or pale skin.

You don't have to overdo eating vegetables and fruits with lots of carotenoids to look and feel younger. Just add more brightly colored fruits and vegetables to your meals, and you could see results in a month.

Don't look old before your time

Fruits, vegetables, lean meat, healthy fats — all these tasty foods can help keep you feeling and looking younger. But there are also foods you should avoid if you don't want to look older than your years.

Stay away from processed foods and soft drinks. Many of them contain damaging phosphates. In fact, soda fountains in the 1950s sold sweet concoctions called "phosphates" — handmade versions of flavored soda pop containing these chemical compounds.

Researchers tested how phosphates behave in the bodies of mice bred to be sensitive to their effects. Turns out phosphates sped up aging in mice, even causing them to die prematurely. High levels of phosphates could also damage your heart and kidneys, and lead to skin and muscle deterioration. Stick to water and other healthy beverages, and keep your skin looking young.

Tomatoes offer triple protection for ageless skin

Did you know that the lycopene in processed tomatoes — including those found in tomato soup and tomato paste — might protect against prostate cancer? It's true, but eating tomatoes can do much more. The high levels of lycopene in this common food may help decrease the appearance of aging on your skin.

Lycopene is an antioxidant carotenoid, so it gets in the way of ultraviolet (UV) radiation from the sun that can damage your skin. Fresh tomatoes and tomato products like juice and soup contain lycopene, but concentrated tomato paste has the highest amount. Here's what it can do for your skin.

Boosts sunburn protection. Sunburn is your skin's cry for help and protection. Covering up with a hat and using sunblock work, but you can also get some protection from the antioxidants in tomato paste.

Researchers in England found that people who ate 5 tablespoons of tomato paste daily had one-third more natural sun protection after just three months. That's about as much defense as using a low SPF sunscreen.

Prevents wrinkles. The top trick to preventing wrinkles and other age-related skin damage is to protect your skin from the sun. When the British researchers looked closely at the skin of the people who had been eating tomato paste, they found higher levels of procollagen. This natural compound gives your skin structure and keeps it looking young and elastic. Other experts have found getting more lycopene in your diet may cut damage to your skin's DNA, reversing the aging process.

Stops skin cancer. A lifetime of exposure to the sun's UV rays can damage your skin's cells, which may lead to skin cancer. But lycopene's antioxidant powers may help protect you from this dangerous consequence of sunbathing.

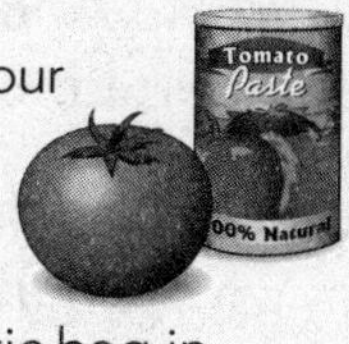

Save the rest of a can of tomato paste when your recipe calls for just a spoonful. Drop the paste by the tablespoon onto a wax paper-lined baking sheet, and freeze until solid. Then store the tomato paste balls in a sealed plastic bag in your freezer. They'll be ready to add to chili or stew.

The researchers warned that eating tomatoes is no substitute for wearing sunscreen, so keep up with your other sun-protection efforts. But when you have the choice, ask for a tomato-based marinara sauce on your spaghetti.

Get super skin with a super juice

A popular brand of pomegranate juice features a stylized heart on the label, hinting at its heart-healthy reputation. Researchers have done a lot to strengthen this reputation, but did you know pomegranate juice may also decrease the appearance of aging on your skin?

Look as young as you feel. Ellagic acid, an antioxidant found in pomegranates, raspberries, and strawberries, protects your skin from collagen breakdown, which can lead to wrinkles. It also fights inflammation and sun damage.

South Korean researchers tested how ellagic acid works using both human skin cells and hairless mice — lab animals with skin that's similar to human skin.

> Pomegranate trees in Versailles, France, are known to be more than 200 years old. It's only right that a long-lasting tree should produce fruit to help you live a long, healthy life.

The skin cells were given a bath of ellagic acid, similar to what happens if you eat lots of berries. Then the cells were exposed to UV radiation, like you get from spending time in the sun. After either 24 or 48 hours of UV exposure, the ellagic acid reduced the destruction of collagen, the protein that gives skin its structure. That's important because a lack of collagen can lead to wrinkles.

Next, the researchers slathered ellagic acid on the skin of hairless mice as part of the experiment. The mice were treated with increasing doses of UV light three times a week for eight weeks. After this extended sunbathing, the mice treated with ellagic acid had less skin wrinkling.

Looking at the results of both studies, the researchers noticed benefits of using this fruity skin care remedy.

Reap additional benefits. While you drink pomegranate juice to keep your outsides looking young, you also do great things for your insides. Research shows that the ellagic acid, vitamin C, and polyphenols in pomegranate juice have these benefits:

- reduce fat stored around your middle — the belly fat that tends to creep up during middle age
- battle high blood pressure and cholesterol
- cut your risk of several types of cancers, including prostate cancer, breast cancer, and cervical cancer
- boost muscle recovery after strenuous exercise
- may fight the inflammation and joint damage of rheumatoid arthritis

Because some of this research was done using pomegranate extract in the form of supplements rather than fresh pomegranate juice, and other studies were done on just a few people, scientists are still investigating exactly how pomegranate might keep you healthy. But even if you enjoy just a fraction of these health benefits, drinking pomegranate juice every day may still be a healthy habit.

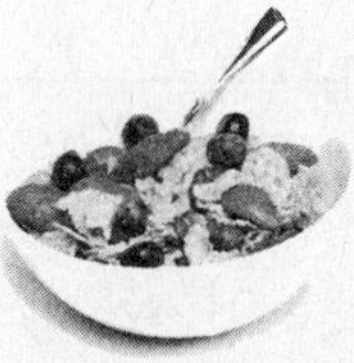

Don't be fooled by a marketing scam. Pictures of colorful fruit on your cereal box can make you think you're getting a healthy breakfast. Not necessarily so — you may be getting little or no fruit. In fact, an image of berries on the box may just mean the cereal contains berry flavoring. So be sure to read the ingredient list to see what's really in your cereal. When you add fresh fruit to your bowl, you know it's really there.

Eat a salad for smoother skin

You don't have to settle for wrinkled skin. Make room for a crispy green salad with just the right dressing, and watch your face grow younger by the bite. This delicious meal is loaded with foods that can fight — and even prevent — wrinkles.

Load up on leafy greens. Researchers in Japan studied the eating habits of 716 women, then examined how old their skin looked. They used the Daniell scale, which assigns a score based on how many wrinkles are on a person's face. The scale ranges from grade I, with basically no wrinkles, to grade VI, with profound wrinkles over most of the face.

Turns out the women who ate more green and yellow vegetables had fewer wrinkles — a good thing, especially if you don't want your age to show all over your face.

Another study found getting more lutein, an antioxidant carotenoid found in abundance in greens like spinach, kale, collards, and lettuce, offers more amazing skin benefits. These researchers looked at women who took lutein supplements — 10 milligrams (mg) a day of lutein along with 0.6 mg zeaxanthin, an antioxidant in many of the same foods as lutein. Some of the women also used cream containing lutein. Taking the supplements worked better than just using the cream, but doing both worked best.

> Instead of using messy over-the-counter ointments to get rid of a stye, reach for a hard-boiled egg. After boiling the egg, let it cool a bit. Then hold the warm egg over your eyelid for several minutes.

Women who got both forms of lutein daily had these improvements in their skin after three months:

- 60 percent better skin hydration, or moisture
- greater protection from sun damage
- 20 percent improvement in skin elasticity

Three cups of fresh spinach in a tasty salad would put you close to the 10 mg lutein the women got from supplements. If that seems like a lot of rabbit food, top your spinach with a couple of hard-boiled eggs or cook up a side dish of kale or collards.

Change your salad dressing. Use a dressing made from olive oil and vinegar instead of a fat-free dressing, and your skin will benefit in two ways.

3 little-known uses for green tea

The antioxidants in green tea make it a great drink to minimize sun damage and speed up the renewal of skin cells. They also can benefit your skin when used topically

- Soothe shaving woes. Next time you end up with nicks and scrapes, sit down to a nice cup of green tea. Then apply the wet tea bag to the cut. The tannic acid in the tea reduces inflammation.
- Soften skin. "Brew" up a refreshing bath by adding green tea bags to the tub while the water runs. Your skin will feel soft and moisturized after a soak.
- Treat acne. Green tea, a natural antibacterial, helps clear up blemishes. Brew up a batch of strong tea, and let it cool. Then use a cotton ball to apply the tea to blemishes. This will calm inflammation and draw out toxins from your skin.

- Adding oil to your salad increases your body's ability to absorb nutrients from the greens. That's one way the monounsaturated fats in olive oil help boost your body's skin-smoothing carotenoid and vitamin E levels.
- Monounsaturated fats, like olive oil, help your skin resist sun damage, a major cause of aging. Studies show foods that contain lots of antioxidants, including vitamin A and vitamin E, help protect skin from dangerous free radicals. Olive oil is one of the best sources of vitamin E.

Ward off wrinkles with vitamin C

Some of your longtime friends never seem to age. Their skin looks smooth and healthy, even as the years fly by. What's their secret? According to researchers in England, it might be an extra orange or grapefruit every morning.

Scientists in Bedford, United Kingdom, looked at results of the first National Health and Nutrition Examination Survey, conducted over a period of four years in the United States. This survey included more than 32,000 men and women, so the researchers had a lot of data to work with.

Women age 40 and older were included in the analysis, which looked for a connection between what they ate and how quickly their skin aged. The women were checked by a dermatologist for wrinkles, thinning, and dryness due to aging. Then the women took a survey to track what they tended to eat on a daily basis. They also answered questions about their exercise habits and other routines.

When the researchers compared the skin evaluations with what the women were eating, they found that those with fewer wrinkles and less dry skin tended to eat more foods high in vitamin C. Citrus fruits and juices were among the women's favorite foods containing this nutrient.

Vitamin C is a powerful antioxidant known for helping your skin build collagen, the protein that keeps skin firm. Vitamin C also protects you from the sun's UV rays, which explains why it's included in products you apply to your skin to prevent wrinkles and sun damage.

Citrus fruits and juices are rich in vitamin C, so enjoy them fresh as often as possible. Top citrus sources of vitamin C include a cup of orange or grapefruit juice, a whole orange or grapefruit, or a cup of mandarin orange slices.

Juicy way to tighten pores

Open your refrigerator and pull out a bottle of skin toner. One spa director recommends using freshly squeezed orange juice on a cotton ball to exfoliate and tone your skin. The juice's vitamin C and alpha hydroxy acids work to tighten pores and prevent blackheads. Rinse off the juice with cool water after a few minutes.

Keep your youthful looks with chocolate

It's no secret that natural compounds in chocolate may benefit your heart and keep your blood flowing smoothly. Now research is finding out how chocolate can help you prevent wrinkles and even avoid skin cancer.

> German researchers found that women who drank a high-flavanol chocolate drink every day had better skin circulation, more protection from sun damage, and improved skin texture and moisture content.

The secret to chocolate's health benefits are the high-antioxidant flavanols found in cocoa beans. Fortunately, the best way to get this type of antioxidant is through your food. You'll also find that green tea and pomegranates are loaded with them. Antioxidants can help protect skin from the damaging effects of the sun's UV radiation, including premature skin aging and skin cancer.

To see how eating chocolate offers protection from the sun, researchers in the United Kingdom tested a high-flavanol chocolate made especially for the study. The chocolate contained more than 600 milligrams (mg) of flavanols in each 20-gram serving, which is about 3/4 of an ounce. They compared this to a low-flavanol chocolate, similar to what people usually eat, that contained less than 30 mg of flavanols per serving.

The 30 people in the study ate a daily serving of either the high-flavanol or low-flavanol chocolate for 12 weeks. Then researchers tested their skin to see how sensitive it was to sunlight using the minimal UVB erythema dose (MED) test. This measures how long it takes for UV light to turn one's skin pink.

Chocolate facial mask

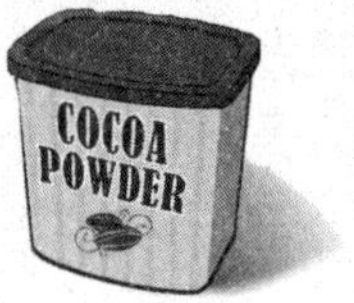

When you've eaten your fill of dark chocolate, give your skin another helping with this nourishing facial mask. There's no need to worry about the calories.

1 tablespoon cocoa powder

1 teaspoon ground oatmeal

2 tablespoons plain yogurt

Blend all the ingredients and massage them onto clean, damp skin. Relax for 15 minutes, then rinse off.

You can also give your whole body a chocolate treat by soaking in a tub fortified with 2 tablespoons cocoa powder and 1/3 cup nonfat dry milk. Be sure to rinse off well to remove all traces of cocoa before you grab a towel.

Folks in the study who ate the high-flavanol chocolate had final MED scores that were more than double their original numbers. That means it took twice as long for a standard dose of UV light to turn their skin pink. In contrast, people who ate regular chocolate didn't have any change in their MED scores after the study.

You can't buy the special high-flavanol chocolate researchers used, but you can look for dark chocolate with a cocoa content of 70 percent or higher to get the best protection.

Clear up eczema by the process of elimination

If you suffer from itchy, dry, scaly, and swollen skin patches on your knees, elbows, hands, feet, and neck, consider whether eczema is the cause. This breakdown of your immune system makes your body overreact to irritants — including things you eat. Experts suggest you may be able to cut down on flare-ups by figuring out which foods trigger the problem.

Try this elimination diet to determine if a food that contains wheat, corn, dairy, eggs, nuts, coffee, or soy is your personal eczema trigger.

- Remove all of the possible culprits from your diet for two weeks. Don't cheat, or you won't know for sure what helps.
- One by one, add each food back into your diet and see whether your skin reacts. Do this by including the food at every meal for three days in a row. You can reintroduce a food to your diet every three days.
- If you have a skin reaction after you start eating a certain food, that's probably the cause of your troubles. Stop eating it for good, and see if your eczema clears up.

Some skin experts suggest attacking eczema by eating foods that can curb inflammation. Try eating more foods high in beta carotene, like carrots and yams, and omega-3 fatty acids, such as flaxseed and oily fish. Give these a try if the elimination diet doesn't uncover a problem food.

Soothe eczema with a remarkable remedy

Want to say so long to itchy, scaly skin? You may be able to get relief by making a tea compress. A small study found that unflavored, black tea helped reduce the itch and severity caused by eczema.

To try it yourself, steep a tea bag in 1 cup of boiling water for 10 minutes. Save the tea bag, but discard this tea. Then steep the used tea bag in another cup of boiling water for 10 minutes. Let it cool, then soak a soft cloth in the tea. Wring it out, then apply the cloth to your eczema for 20 minutes. Remove, and apply moisturizer.

Lock in moisture with a natural supplement

When you've had it with smearing on lotions and creams to calm your dry, itchy skin, look to wheat extract oil to moisturize your skin from the inside out.

These capsules are a rich source of ceramides, a fatty substance found naturally in your skin that binds cells together to keep in moisture. Researchers tested the supplements by giving them to women with dry skin. Half the women took 350 milligrams (mg) of Lipowheat, a form of wheat extract oil, daily for three months. The other half took a sugar pill.

For a topical source of these natural fatty compounds, look for ceramides on the ingredient list of super-moisturizing lotions.

At the start and end of the study, the women and dermatologists both analyzed the skin on their arms, legs, and face to see how dry, rough, and red it appeared. Women who took the wheat extract oil had better-hydrated skin by the end of the study. In fact, these women noticed the improvement even though they didn't know which pills they had been taking.

You can buy capsules containing wheat extract oil from brands like Life Extension and Swanson. Check your local drugstore or grocery, or shop online.

HEALTH ALERT!

Skip the beer, and you may be able to avoid psoriasis. Researchers followed nearly 83,000 women in the Nurses' Health Study II for 14 years, tracking whether they drank alcohol and if they developed psoriasis. This itchy skin condition related to immune system problems was already linked with alcohol, but the researchers wanted to see if what women drank made a difference.

They found that women who drank five or more beers a week were nearly twice as likely to develop psoriasis compared with women who didn't drink alcohol. Drinking light beer, wine, or liquor didn't seem to raise their psoriasis risk. The experts suspect the gluten in the barley used to brew beer might be at fault. Light beer is made with less barley.

Bone-building nutrients keep skin safe

Calcium and vitamin D are good for more than just protecting your bones. They may also help prevent skin cancer if you are at high risk.

Keep supplements on your radar. Researchers in California looked at the results of a large study that followed 36,000 women for more than seven years. Half the women in the trial took calcium and vitamin D supplements every day, while half took a placebo. The researchers checked to see which of the women developed skin cancer during that time.

For most of the women, taking supplements didn't make a difference in their skin cancer risk. But for those who had already suffered from a nonmelanoma cancer — squamous cell carcinoma or basal cell carcinoma — supplements made a big difference. Their risk of developing the more deadly melanoma was 57 percent lower than for women taking the placebo.

The women took a relatively low dose of supplements — just 1,000 milligrams of calcium and 400 international units of vitamin D. You could get nearly that much calcium from drinking three glasses of skim milk and that much vitamin D from 3.5 ounces of wild-caught salmon.

Tasty meal for skin protection

Enjoy a glass of wine with a fish dinner regularly, and you may steer clear of skin cancer. Researchers in Australia looked at what people ate and how many of them developed actinic keratoses — small, rough areas related to spending time in the sun. Some actinic keratoses can become cancerous.

The researchers found fewer of these lesions among people who ate oily fish at least once a week and drank half a glass of wine daily. Omega-3 fatty acids in fish — especially oily varieties like sardines and trout — and resveratrol and other antioxidants in wine may be responsible for the protective effect of this meal.

You don't want to overdo drinking alcohol or eating fish, but this research shows another way to protect your skin.

Don't shun the sun. It's no surprise that people who have already suffered a bout with skin cancer tend to avoid spending time in the sun. One result? Research shows that these folks are three times more likely to be deficient in vitamin D than other people. That's bad news, since sunlight is a major source of vitamin D, which helps keep you safe from heart disease, certain cancers, and immune disorders like multiple sclerosis.

If you're not at risk for skin cancer, get out in the sunshine. Your body can easily make vitamin D from the sun's ultraviolet rays. Experts recommend five to 30 minutes of sunlight — without wearing sunscreen — at least twice a week on your face, hands, and legs. If you stay out in the sun longer, apply a sunscreen with an SPF of at least 30.

Make low-fat your go-to dairy. Be sure to choose low-fat dairy for your vitamin D and calcium. Researchers in Australia surveyed more than 1,400 people to see what foods they ate. Then they tracked how many of them developed skin cancer over 11 years.

It turns out that those who ate more full-fat dairy, along with red meat, processed meat, fat, processed grains, and sweetened beverages, suffered more squamous cell carcinomas than those who ate a more produce-based diet. People who ate vegetables, fruits, unprocessed grains, low-fat dairy, and fish had a lower risk of skin cancer. The difference was even greater for people who had previously had skin cancer.

Coffee every day keeps cancer at bay

Don't feel guilty when you pour yourself a third cup of coffee. Your daily caffeine habit just might help prevent the most common type of skin cancer, basal cell carcinoma.

About 3.6 million new cases of basal cell carcinoma are diagnosed each year in the United States. It accounts for about 80 percent of skin cancers.

Did you know?

Contact skin allergies may be a sign of greater protection against some forms of cancer.

Researchers in Denmark found that people who suffer allergic reactions from touching certain materials like acetone, nickel, or cobalt may have "hyperimmunity." That means their immune systems are extra protective against outside invaders, in this case causing a skin rash. The researchers then discovered that people with skin allergies had a lower risk of developing nonmelanoma skin cancer and breast cancer.

More than 10 percent of people in the United States suffer from contact allergies. If that includes you, take heart knowing you may be protected against a bigger ill.

Researchers used information from the massive Nurses' Health Study and Health Professionals Follow-Up Study to examine coffee drinking habits and cases of basal cell carcinoma, squamos cell carcinoma, and melanoma.

The researchers found that women who drank at least 3 cups of coffee a day — caffeinated coffee, not the decaffeinated kind — were 20 percent less likely to develop basal cell carcinoma than people who drank less than 1 cup a month. Men who drank at least 3 cups of coffee a day were also less likely to get skin cancer, but their risk was just 9 percent lower than people who drank less than a cup a month.

The experts aren't sure how coffee protects, but they think the caffeine may kill off certain precancerous cells that have been damaged by the sun's ultraviolet light and "gone rogue." Caffeine seems to kill them before they can become cancerous.

Previous research found similar results among a different group of women. Those scientists suggested that caffeine's antioxidant effects might make cells less likely to become cancerous.

No matter the explanation, experts caution coffee drinkers to continue protecting themselves against skin cancer by avoiding sunburn and having a doctor look at any suspicious skin growths.

Stay tick-free with clove oil

You can repel ticks when you hike and come out of the woods bite-free if you apply a bit of clove oil first.

Experts found certain essential oils, including clove, citronella, and lily of the valley, work as well as the insecticide chemical DEET at repelling ticks. The natural ingredient eugenol is what makes clove oil so powerful, making it effective against scabies mites as well as ticks.

Don't put concentrated clove oil directly on your skin, since it can be irritating. Dilute two drops of clove oil in a tablespoon of olive oil. Then apply it directly to areas of exposed skin before you go hiking. Wash it off once you're back inside.

Pick a 'berry' good nail solution

You can stop drinking gelatin powders and taking calcium pills to make your fingernails strong. There's no good research to show these supplements will help. But there's one nutrient that may help cure brittle nails — biotin.

Your pantry also contains a great cuticle treatment. Apply a dab of olive oil to your nail beds to moisturize the cuticles.

Animal experts found they could treat horses and pigs with hoof problems by feeding them supplements of biotin, a B complex vitamin. That discovery made researchers wonder if biotin could strengthen people's nails, too. Here's what they found — you can get rid of brittle nails when you get the nutrients you need naturally.

Toss hand lotion that's thin enough to run. When its high water content evaporates, brittle nails are left unprotected. Pick a thick cream that keeps moisture in.

Three studies on biotin supplements as a treatment for brittle fingernails all found the vitamin may help. One trial found that people who took biotin supplements had less nail splitting and enjoyed nails that were as much as 25 percent thicker. The other two trials showed at least some improvement in up to 91 percent of the people taking biotin. Those are incredible results.

If you don't want to take supplements, you can get biotin from eating meat, poultry, eggs, and dairy foods. But you may prefer a fruitier source of biotin — strawberries. They're high in biotin and easy to brew into a cup of wonderful nail-strengthening tea.

Strawberry tea

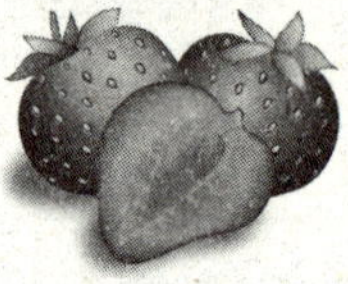

2 cups water

1 tea bag, strawberry tea or green tea, decaffeinated

1/2 cup sliced strawberries, fresh or frozen

1 tablespoon honey or sugar substitute

Bring water to a boil in a saucepan over medium heat. Remove from the heat. Add the tea bag, strawberries, and sweetener. Cover the pan, and let steep for five minutes.

Strain out the berries and pour into two cups. Enjoy with a friend.

Feed your hair from the inside out

Some common causes of hair loss have nothing to do with aging and everything to do with what you eat. You can give your hair everything it needs to grow healthy and strong just by eating a bowl of clam chowder. This cold-weather treat is loaded with protein, iron, and B vitamins.

Pack in the protein. Starving your body, especially of protein, can bring on a kind of hair loss called telogen effluvium. This type of hair thinning occurs all over your head rather than in patches.

Researchers in France looked at how eating patterns might be causing hair loss among a group of young people 20 to 35 years old. They compared their diets to a similar group who had no trouble with hair loss. Turns out how much protein they ate was the only big difference.

Clams might not be your first thought for a protein-rich food, but they're packed with this muscle-building nutrient. A 3-ounce serving boasts 22 grams of protein. That's a big part of what your body needs in a day.

Pump it up with iron. It's also possible to suffer from hair loss if you don't eat enough important minerals, including iron and zinc. A 3.5 ounce serving of cooked clams has some zinc, but it's a real iron powerhouse with 35 percent of the iron you need in a day.

Research has been mixed concerning which types of hair loss might be affected by a lack of iron. But if you're a woman suffering from thinning hair, ask your doctor about a blood test to check your iron and red blood cell levels.

Be sure to include B complex. Experts also say a lack of B complex vitamins, including biotin, folate, and vitamin B12, may contribute to thinning hair. You'll get a bounty of B12 from clams, but you may also want to ask your doctor about taking a B-complex vitamin to speed up your hair's regrowth.

There's a history of strong feelings in New England about how clam chowder should be made. Lawmakers in Maine in 1939 introduced a bill making it illegal to add tomatoes to the chowder, while folks in Rhode Island typically use tomatoes. Happily for your health, you have a choice.

A 1 cup serving of New England-style clam chowder, the white kind, has 154 calories and 5 grams of fat. That's because it's made with milk or cream. Pick a healthier version by asking for the tomato-based Manhattan style — just 2 grams of fat and 75 calories per cup.

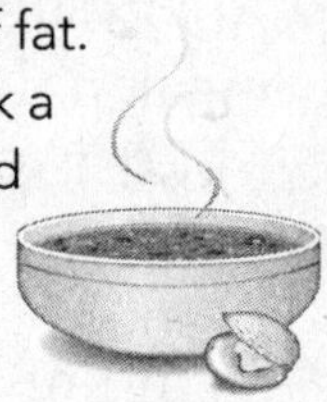

Soothe your scalp with herbs

Skip those smelly medicated shampoos advertised for a dry, itchy scalp. You can keep your scalp feeling clean and refreshed with one of these herbal treatments.

Relieve the itch with rosemary. Blend together 4 tablespoons of olive oil with 4 tablespoons of honey, and mix in 3 drops of rosemary essential oil. Heat the mixture in a double boiler until it's warm — not hot. Then massage it into your damp hair and scalp. Let it sit for 30 minutes, then wash out.

Rosemary is traditionally used to kill bacteria and funguses and treat poor circulation. Never eat rosemary essential oil, since it can be toxic.

Revive with mint and parsley. If it's that tingly, cool sensation you crave, try using this refreshing toner.

Chop up a handful each of fresh parsley and mint leaves and place them in a glass bowl. Boil 1/2 cup of water and pour it over the herbs to steep. Let the mixture cool, strain out the leaves, and add 1/2 cup of witch hazel. After you shampoo, apply the toner to your scalp with a cotton ball, and massage it in.

Tame dandruff with salmon

Dandruff may not be bad for your health, but it sure can put a damper on your looks. And it's no small problem — millions of Americans suffer from this scaly, itchy scalp condition. Dandruff may get worse during times of stress, cold weather, when you color your hair, or use too much styling product.

Nutritional deficiencies — not eating enough B vitamins and omega-3 fatty acids — can also make dandruff worse. That may be especially true if you tend to have dry skin. Add a serving of salmon to your weekly dinner rotation, and you'll boost your levels of these important nutrients.

Omega-3 fatty acids. Great sources of this healthy fat include flaxseed oil, canola oil, and a variety of deep-water fish like herring and mackerel. But fresh salmon is the real winner when it comes to being a tasty source of omega-3 fatty acids, containing nearly 2 grams in a 3.5-ounce serving.

B vitamins. This group of water-soluble vitamins, including thiamin, niacin, vitamin B6, and vitamin B12, help keep your skin and hair healthy. That same serving of salmon provides you with a good amount of those two important nutrients. You can also get B vitamins from egg yolks, bananas, nuts, dark leafy greens, whole grains, soybeans, and avocados.

Did you know?

Got embarrassing dandruff? Get rid of it with these two home remedies. Best of all, you probably already have the ingredients in your pantry.

- Vinegar. Mix equal parts of water and apple cider vinegar in a spray bottle. Before applying, do a patch test on the back of your hand. If there's no reaction, massage the mixture into your scalp. Let it sit for a few minutes. Then rinse out, and shampoo.

- Salt. Sprinkle some sea salt near the roots of your hair. Then massage the salt into your scalp with wet fingers to exfoliate the area. Follow with a regular shampooing.

Tendonitis & bursitis

Spicy solution for painful inflammation

Need to soothe tendonitis pain in a hurry? Eat some curry. That's because Indian curries and many other ethnic foods feature the spice turmeric — and turmeric contains a powerful polyphenol called curcumin.

A team of British and German researchers discovered that curcumin, which gives turmeric its distinctive yellow color, helps suppress inflammation in tendonitis.

This painful condition occurs when tendons, the dense connective tissue between muscles and bones, become injured through overuse. Tendonitis, or tendon inflammation, often affects joints in your shoulders, knees, elbows, hips, heels, and wrists, leaving these areas tender and sore.

To deal with the pain and reduce inflammation, you can always take nonsteroidal anti-inflammatory drugs (NSAIDs), like aspirin or ibuprofen. But these remedies often come with unpleasant side effects, including ulcers, nausea, heartburn, fatigue, diarrhea, and constipation. This study suggests that curcumin could be a natural, safer alternative.

In the study, scientists tested curcumin on tendon cells. They found that curcumin interrupts a key signaling pathway that triggers inflammation. Specifically, curcumin inhibits the activation of Nuclear Factor-kB (NF-kB) by pro-inflammatory messengers called interleukins. That's important because if NF-kB becomes activated, it can spark even more inflammation.

Because of its anti-inflammatory powers, curcumin may also help people with other conditions involving inflammation, such as arthritis. Although curcumin isn't a miracle cure, the research on it has been quite consistent. So be sure to add some delicious turmeric to your diet.

You can find powdered turmeric in your supermarket's spice aisle. Sprinkle some into a stir-fry, or experiment with other ways to cook with this flavorful spice. You can also enjoy a healthy helping of turmeric in curry dishes at Indian or Thai restaurants. Think of it as a way to treat your taste buds while soothing your tendonitis.

Basic tips to battle bursitis

Injuries like tendonitis and bursitis — inflammation of the bursa, small fluid-filled sacs that cushion tissues near joints — can occur when you push your body too hard. Make sure your exercise routine doesn't put you at risk.

- Warm up before workouts by walking in place or pedaling in a low gear for a few minutes. Do the same thing to cool down until your breathing and heart rate return to normal.
- Joints, muscles, and tendons become less flexible as you age, so they benefit from a gentle stretch after you have warmed up.
- Don't perform the same exercises every day. Using different muscle groups helps you avoid injuries.
- Take frequent breaks when performing repetitive tasks, like vacuuming or raking leaves. Take a day off when you feel an ache. Don't try to push through the pain.
- Knee and elbow pads can help cushion your joints from pressure.

If you do develop bursitis, apply an ice pack for 10 to 15 minutes, as often as twice an hour, for three days. Then switch to a heating pad.

Urinary incontinence

Eat to beat the bathroom blues

Watch what you eat and drink, and you may solve the problem of a leaky bladder.

Eating the wrong mix of fats may contribute to inflammation and problems with the lining of your blood vessels, experts say. Some research suggests these changes may even cause urinary problems. In fact, one study found that women who ate more saturated fats than polyunsaturated fats (PUFAs) had a higher risk of developing incontinence — and it was more likely to be severe.

Saturated fats are found in meats, dairy foods like milk and cheese, and oils like palm oil that are solid at room temperature. Foods high in PUFAs include fish, walnuts, flaxseed, and liquid oils like corn oil, safflower oil, soybean oil, and sunflower oil.

Women who ate equal amounts of saturated fats and PUFAs had less risk of incontinence and severe incontinence than women who ate three times as much saturated fat as PUFAs. But that's not all. Women who cut back on calories also had less severe incontinence and were less likely to develop the problem in the first place. In fact, the researchers suggest that up to 70 percent of the cases in their study could have been prevented by eating a healthy diet and following these guidelines.

- Eat no more than one-and-a-half times as much saturated fat as PUFAs. Replacing some servings of meats and dairy with fish, nuts, or nut butters is a good place to start. Also, be sure to check for saturated fats on the labels of packaged foods before you buy them.

- Place a healthy limit on the number of calories you eat each day. Check with your doctor before you cut many calories.
- Aim for a normal-weight body mass index (BMI) of 18.5 to 24.9.

In addition to these changes, experiment to find any trigger foods or drinks that may contribute to incontinence. Eliminate one or two of the following at a time, for two weeks, to see if you improve. You can add back foods if you don't notice any changes in your symptoms.

- alcoholic beverages
- citrus fruits and juices
- caffeinated drinks and decaffeinated coffee
- caffeine-free carbonated drinks
- chocolate
- spicy foods
- artificial sweeteners, sugar, and honey
- tomato-based drinks and foods
- milk and milk-based foods

Did you know?

A little sunshine might do your bladder good. A study found that women who have the lowest blood levels of vitamin D have a higher risk of incontinence. But that risk goes down as vitamin D levels rise.

Researchers think a lack of this critical vitamin may limit the strength of pelvic muscles, raising your odds of incontinence. Your body makes vitamin D when sunlight touches your skin, so pump up your levels by spending more time outdoors. You should also focus on eating foods rich in vitamin D. Good choices include fatty fish like salmon as well as vitamin-D-fortified cereals and dairy products.

Vision loss

Keep peepers healthy with leafy greens

Odds are, Popeye never got cataracts. Whether it's canned, frozen, or freshly cooked, spinach packs a punch when it comes to protecting your eyesight. This leafy green boasts loads of lutein and zeaxanthin, two antioxidants your eyes can't do without.

The more lutein and zeaxanthin you have in your blood, the lower your risk of nuclear cataracts, says a study out of Finland. Seniors between the ages of 61 and 80 with the most lutein and zeaxanthin in their blood were about 40 percent less likely to develop this type of cataract.

Sunlight, smoking, normal aging, and diabetes all damage the lens of your eye over a lifetime. They create free radicals that attack the proteins in your lenses. Fortunately, your body can fight back with powerful antioxidants.

Healthy eyes contain lots of lutein and zeaxanthin. These two plant compounds neutralize free radicals and filter out blue light, the kind that does the most damage to your eyes. Sometimes, though, free radicals overwhelm these natural defenses. That's how cataracts develop.

You refill your eyes' stockpile of antioxidants every time you eat foods like spinach. Your body flushes these compounds out of your bloodstream in a few days, however, so eat a steady supply to keep your stores high.

Studies suggest you need at least 6 milligrams (mg) a day of lutein and zeaxanthin combined to help prevent cataracts. Getting these nutrients couldn't be easier. Just 1 cup of boiled spinach packs 20 mg of these sight-saving antioxidants. Other leafy greens, like kale and collard greens, will do the job, too. Keep your vision eagle-eye sharp by choosing the right foods. Read on for more of the best — and worst — foods for your eyesight.

Did you know?

Smoking depletes your natural stores of lutein and zeaxanthin, which damages the lenses in your eyes. And taking corticosteroids by mouth or inhaled through the nose increases your chances of developing nuclear cataracts. Eating more lutein and zeaxanthin could help offset the harm done by both.

Nature's all-natural cataract preventers

A lifetime spent loading your plate with red meat could make you more likely to develop vision problems, such as cataracts. But if you switch up your meals to feature more fish or go vegetarian, you may be able to keep your vision clear.

Vegetables are top sources of eye-protecting antioxidants, including vitamins C and E and the compounds lutein and zeaxanthin. Animal foods, on the other hand, contain lots of saturated fat, which seems to raise your risk of cataracts.

Seniors in particular could benefit from cutting back on meat. British researchers looked at the eating habits of 27,000 people, and then followed up to see who developed cataracts. The results were astounding. Compared to seniors who ate more than one serving of meat every day, those who pared meat from their diet were much less likely to develop cataracts. (See graph.)

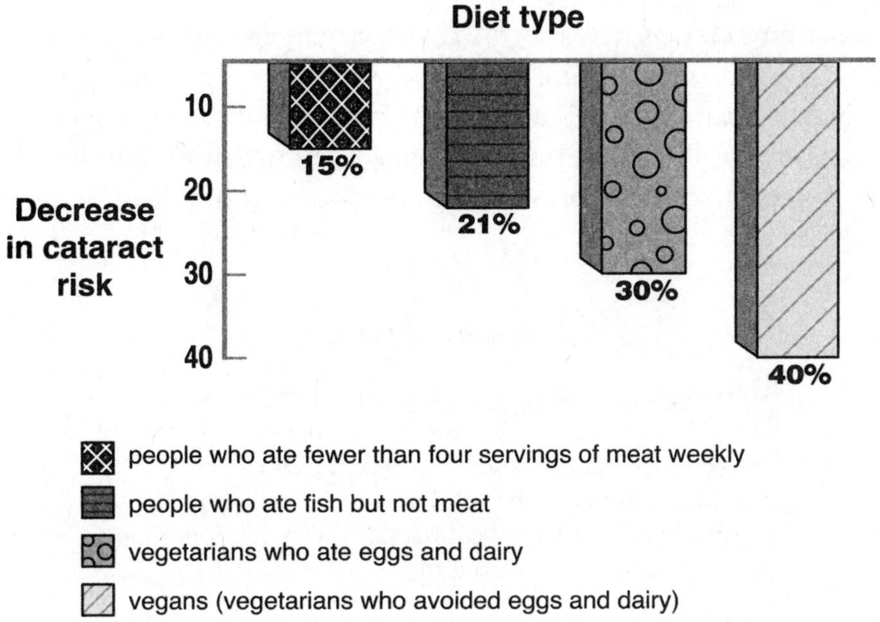

You can cut meat and saturated fat from your diet without feeling deprived. Here are some painless ways to make the switch.

Beef up on beans. If you decide to give up meat, make sure you eat two servings of beans and legumes each day. They're an important source of protein for vegetarians. This includes the typical black beans and pinto beans, but don't forget about hummus made from chickpeas or soybeans served as edamame.

Get meaty with mushrooms. They give you the texture of meat without the fat. Plus, they're the only plant source of vitamin D. Grill a portobello mushroom instead of a hamburger. Place it in a hamburger bun and top with lettuce and tomatoes for a meat-free summer lunch. On taco nights, try chopped mushrooms in place of ground meat.

Oil your pans. Stir-fry vegetables with canola oil instead of butter. Grease baking pans with nonstick vegetable spray instead of butter, margarine, or shortening.

Bake smarter. When a recipe calls for margarine or butter in baked goodies, substitute applesauce, cottage cheese, pureed bananas, prunes, or garbanzo beans instead. This swap works especially well in cakes, brownies, breads, and muffins. For one idea, see "Black bean brownies" in the *Heart disease* chapter.

Did you know?

Prevent cataracts and strengthen your eyesight with tuna. The omega-3 fatty acids in this fish can help protect your eyesight. A study found that people who got at least 500 milligrams (mg) of this nutrient daily were 42 percent less likely to get cataracts. You'll find more than that in 3 ounces of albacore tuna.

Omega-3s also fight age-related macular degeneration (AMD), a condition in which central vision deteriorates. Researchers found that women who got around 330 mg of omega-3s a day had a 38% lower risk of developing AMD than those who averaged 80 mg.

Fine-tune your focus with these natural vision savers

Collard greens are a Southern staple that everyone should learn to love. The link between its nutrients and the health of your eyesight is indisputable.

Leafy greens like collards and kale are top sources of two plant compounds — lutein and zeaxanthin — that preserve your vision. They're the only two carotenoids found inside both the lens of your eye and the macula.

As natural antioxidants, they:

- snuff out dangerous free radical compounds, guarding the macula from sight-stealing oxidative damage.
- absorb blue light, the kind that does the most harm to your retina.

This may explain why, in one study, people who had the most lutein and zeaxanthin in their retinas were 82 percent less likely to develop macular degeneration than those with the least.

Eat more and see better. You can boost the amount of these compounds in your eyes without resorting to drugs or medicine of any kind. Simply eat more leafy greens. Your body will deliver these nutrients to your eyes, which may help improve your eyesight without the need for surgery or glasses. In one study, men with macular degeneration who added 5 ounces of spinach to their diet at least four days a week saw significant improvements in their vision in one year.

Pay attention to eye color. People with light-colored eyes should make an extra effort to eat more lutein and zeaxanthin by loading up on collards and other green, leafy vegetables. Light colored eyes can let in 100 times more light than dark brown eyes. Add to that, people with blue, gray, green, and hazel eyes have lower levels of lutein and zeaxanthin in their maculas to begin with. This combination leaves them especially vulnerable to vision damage.

Cook your leafy greens to get the most sight-saving nutrients. They contain more lutein and zeaxanthin than the raw versions. Cooking seems to break down plant cells just enough to release more of these protective compounds.

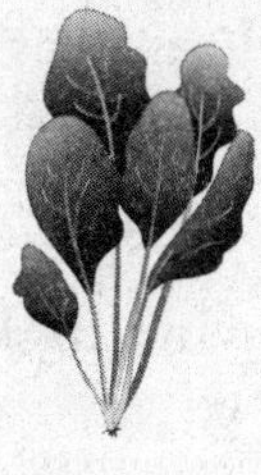

Beware of smoking. This habit is a proven risk factor for macular degeneration. Smoking also depletes your eyes of lutein and zeaxanthin. If you're a smoker, you'll need to get more foods like kale, collards, turnips, and spinach.

Supercharge your salad

Think vegetables are good for you? They're not nearly as healthy without a dash of olive oil. You could protect your sight from macular degeneration and cataracts simply by tossing a bit on your salad.

The heart-healthy fat in olive oil boosts the nutrition of the other ingredients. You see, your body can't absorb carotenoids like lutein, zeaxanthin, or beta carotene without fat. It's that simple. People who ate an antioxidant-rich salad topped with fat-free dressing absorbed next to no lycopene or carotene. Reduced-fat dressings helped a little, but people got the most nutrients when they used full-fat dressing.

Opt for extra virgin olive oil instead of commercial salad dressing. Top each serving of salad with at least 1 teaspoon of olive oil.

Offbeat berry may prevent blindness

A simple berry could save your eyesight from the ravages of age-related macular degeneration (AMD). Bilberries, a close relative of blueberries, possess some potent antioxidants called anthocyanins.

Bilberries have been used to treat eye conditions for years, from improving night vision to preventing cataracts and glaucoma.

In fact, British fighter pilots in World War II reported better night vision when they ate bilberry jam.

AMD is the latest eye disease that may benefit from these humble berries. In a study on animals prone to vision problems, 7 in 10 developed cataracts or macular degeneration when they were fed a regular diet. Among those fed bilberry-enriched food, none developed these conditions.

The anthocyanins in bilberries seem to stop your body from pumping out free radicals. When free radicals build up in the retina, they trigger inflammation. This condition, in turn, damages the eye cells that receive incoming light and pass it along to the brain. If the inflammation goes on long enough, these light-sensing cells can break down. Bilberries, however, may protect these all-important cells from the ravages of inflammation.

Don't fret if you can't find bilberries. Blueberries make a great substitute. They're another top-notch source of anthocyanins. Some research suggests blueberries themselves may improve vision. Rabbits fed blueberries suffered less damage to their retinas from bright light.

This common fruit protects your heart and veins, too. One study found that eating just one serving of blueberries a week made people less likely to develop high blood pressure. That, in turn, helps prevent strokes, heart disease, heart attacks, and heart failure. So whether you like them fresh, frozen, canned, or jellied, make blueberries part of your everyday diet.

Save your eyesight with budget-friendly fish

Eating fatty fish on a regular basis could protect women from losing their sight to age-related macular degeneration (AMD).

Out of more than 38,000 women, those who ate at least one serving of fish each week had a whopping 42 percent lower risk of AMD than women who ate fish less than once a month. These weren't fancy seafood dinners, either. Most of the benefit came from eating canned tuna, salmon, and sardines. That means saving your eyesight doesn't have to break the bank.

Quench the burn. Fish is a top source of two specific fats — EPA and DHA. Both are omega-3 fatty acids known for squashing inflammation. Experts think that's one way they block AMD from developing.

Your body uses omega-3s and omega-6s, to make compounds called eicosanoids. Eicosanoids made from omega-6s cause inflammation, whereas eicosanoids made from omega-3s generally don't. Inflammation plays a major role in the development of AMD. By soothing it, fish fats may help prevent this disease.

Dairy does double duty

Milk does more than build strong bones. Studies show it may also safeguard your sight. Women under the age of 75 were half as likely to develop early-stage macular degeneration if they had relatively high levels of vitamin D in their blood.

Vitamin D may block inflammation from damaging delicate parts of the eye in the early stages of age-related macular degeneration (AMD). Supplements and food sources of this vitamin — such as milk, fish, and fortified cereal — lowered AMD risk, but sunlight did not.

Your doctor can test your vitamin D levels during your next physical. The magic number in this study was 38 nanomols per liter (nmol/L). Higher levels didn't seem to offer any additional protection.

Guard your blood vessels. AMD has a lot in common with heart disease. Scientists suspect they even share some of the same causes, including inflammation. It makes sense, then, that the same fish fats that guard your heart also fight AMD. The unsaturated fish fats EPA and DHA help prevent hardening of the arteries and the formation of dangerous blood clots in vessels, and they may help improve blood flow to your eyes.

So start serving up more fish, even if it comes from a can. Make a point to eat two servings every week for strong vision that will last a lifetime.

All-natural oil relieves dry eyes

Artificial tears work as a stopgap for soothing dry eyes, but they only mask symptoms. They don't clear up the underlying cause of this condition. The oil in flaxseeds might.

Flaxseeds are rich in omega-3 fatty acids, a type of heart-healthy unsaturated fat. Most people don't get nearly enough. They do, however, get more than enough omega-6 fats. While these two types of fat are related, they have very different effects in your body. An overload of omega-6s may cause inflammation, and can even lead to heart disease and stroke.

Find the right balance. Eating more omega-3s helps counteract these negative effects. Experts suggest that for every 4 grams of omega-6s in your diet, you should try to eat 1 gram of omega-3s. Unfortunately, most folks in developed countries like the United States miss that mark by a long shot, getting 20 grams or more of omega-6s for every 1 gram of omega-3s. That's because people eat too much meat and processed foods, which tend to be high in omega-6s, and too little fish, flaxseed, and canola oil, which are rich in omega-3s.

Heed the warning. Your eyes could be trying to warn you that you're way out of whack in the fats you eat each day. Women who get a healthy balance of omega-3s to omega-6s are less likely to suffer from dry eye syndrome. In one study, people who ate the most omega-3s were 20 percent less likely to develop dry eyes.

Take steps to change. Omega-3 fatty acids from flaxseed and fish fight dry eyes in four ways by:

- restoring the natural layer of fat that keeps your eyes lubricated.
- cooling inflammation that contributes to dry eye syndrome.
- helping your body produce more tears naturally.
- preventing tears from evaporating.

Flaxseed is one of the best sources for these vision-friendly fats. It packs three times more omega-3s than omega-6s. Shop for fresh, whole flaxseeds, since they'll keep longer than ground ones. Your body absorbs the nutrients from ground seeds much better than from whole. So grind the seeds yourself in a coffee grinder as you need them.

Sprinkle ground flaxseed on hot cereal, vegetables, or any other dish. You can also buy flaxseed oil to drizzle on salads. Never cook with it, though. Refrigerate the oil, and keep ground flaxseed in an airtight container in the freezer.

Weight gain

A great reason to drink chocolate milk

Got belly fat? Exercise regularly, cut back on calories — and don't forget to drink your chocolate milk. This sweet beverage is more than a tasty treat. It also gives you a boost in the battle of the bulge. Studies highlight how low-fat chocolate milk, along with exercise, can help make that belly disappear.

Lose fat and build muscle. Canadian researchers found that a high-protein, high-dairy diet plus exercise equals success. The Improving Diet, Exercise, and Lifestyle (IDEAL) for Women Study featured 90 overweight or obese women ages 19 to 45, split into three groups.

One group ate more dairy and protein and fewer carbohydrates than the others. That group also drank Splenda-sweetened 1-percent chocolate milk twice a day, once right after exercising and again at least five hours before or after exercising.

At the end of the 16-week study, which included both aerobic exercise and weightlifting, this group lost about the same amount of weight as the other groups — but they lost more fat, built more muscle, and had greater increases in strength than the other groups.

Credit likely goes to calcium and other components of dairy products, including milk proteins that help trim fat while maintaining muscle during weight loss.

Banish cravings with these 3 foods

Just a little fat with lunch might help you avoid becoming a lot fatter by dinner. Eating a slice of avocado, a dash of olive oil, or a handful of nuts with lunch will make you less hungry for the rest of the day.

Avocados, olive oil, and nuts are full of monounsaturated fat (MUFA), and research shows a particular MUFA called oleic acid causes a chemical reaction that calms hunger pangs.

Oleic acid prompts the small intestine to produce the hunger-fighting compound oleoylethanolamide (OEA). In turn, OEA trips the switch that makes your digestive tract tell your brain it's full. The result — you feel full for longer, which can help stop snack cravings between meals.

Help your body recover. University of Texas researchers had similar results. In a pair of studies, one involving 10 experienced cyclists and the other involving 32 untrained people, chocolate milk worked its magic.

Drinking low-fat chocolate milk after a cycling workout improves endurance and performance, builds muscles, and reduces fat. Results were better among those who drank this beverage compared to those who drank a carbohydrate drink with no protein or a no-calorie placebo beverage.

Turns out chocolate milk provides the perfect combination of carbohydrates and protein to help your body recover after a workout. The carbohydrates help replace glycogen, which your body burns for energy, while the protein helps maintain muscle mass and prevent muscle breakdown. Flavonoids in chocolate milk could also have a beneficial effect.

Make it part of your workout. Keep in mind that these studies were funded by groups like the Dairy Farmers of Canada, the U.S. Dairy Research Institute, the National Dairy Council, and the National Fluid Milk Processor Promotion Board. But that doesn't mean the results aren't valid.

Consider making low-fat chocolate milk part of your exercise routine. For best results, drink a glass of this beverage within 20 to 30 minutes after your workout. You just might sip your way to a slimmer belly.

Thanks to low-fat chocolate milk and other fat-busting foods, a flat belly can be yours. Read more of this chapter to discover other foods that can help you achieve it.

Bowl over belly fat with cereal

Looking for a secret way to naturally block out calories from foods? You can trick your body into losing weight by adding high-fiber foods to your diet. Your body takes a long time to digest them, so you feel full for longer. That means you'll be less likely to snack between meals.

And because high-fiber foods like fruits and veggies tend to be lower in calories than processed fare, you'll be able to eat more and end up weighing less. Plus all that roughage may help prevent type 2 diabetes and cardiovascular disease.

One of the best ways to make sure you're getting your daily fiber fix is to eat more cereal. So check out what the research says, and learn how easy it is to sneak cereal into your diet each day.

Fight back with fiber. A large European study tracked the eating habits of more than 89,000 adults, ages 20 to 78, for an average of six-and-a-half years. Researchers found that total fiber — but especially cereal fiber — was linked to weight loss and a slimmer waistline.

The changes were small, but statistically significant. Over a year, eating 10 grams of cereal fiber a day resulted in weight loss of 77 grams, or about an eighth of a pound. It also shrunk waist size by 0.10 centimeters, or about 0.04 inches.

Cereal fiber doesn't just refer to breakfast cereal. Other sources include rice, pasta, breads, biscuits, crackers, and other products made of flour, especially whole-grain flour.

Opt for oats. Here's some cheery news for Cheerios lovers. More of this whole-grain oat cereal means less belly fat and healthier hearts. Those are the benefits folks get when they add this easy-to-find and delicious food to their diets.

In a 12-week study of overweight and obese people with high cholesterol, those who ate about 3 cups of oat cereal a day fared better than the low-fiber control group. Both groups were encouraged to limit foods high in calories and fat, practice portion control, and exercise regularly as part of the diet program.

While both groups lost similar amounts of weight, the oat cereal group significantly reduced their waist size by 3.3 centimeters, or 1.3 inches. They also lowered their bad LDL cholesterol level by 8.7 percent and total cholesterol by 5.4 percent.

These positive results probably stem from beta glucan, a type of soluble fiber found in oats. People in the Cheerios group got 3 grams of beta glucan each day. But by eating cereal and milk, they also boosted their intake of calcium, magnesium, potassium, and vitamin D.

Swap your snacks. Cereal isn't just for breakfast. If you get the munchies in the evening, swap your usual nighttime snack for a

> ### Beware of midmorning munchies
>
> Timing is everything — at least when it comes to snacking. Research suggests that snacking between breakfast and lunch could hamper your weight loss efforts.
>
> In a study of 123 dieting women ages 50 to 75, those who reported snacking between 10:30 a.m. and 11:30 a.m. lost less weight than those who didn't. Midmorning snackers lost only 7 percent of their body weight during the yearlong study, while those who didn't snack before lunch lost more than 11 percent.
>
> But that doesn't mean snacking is bad. The study also found that afternoon snackers ate more fruits and vegetables, and that those who ate two or more snacks a day got more fiber. A nutritious, low-calorie snack can help hold you over during breaks between meals so that you don't make poor food choices at mealtime. Just make sure you only snack when you're hungry and not out of habit or boredom.

bowl of cereal. A British study found that this simple strategy helped overweight snackers shed pounds and lower their daily calorie intake.

Here are some other ways to sneak extra cereal fiber — from breakfast cereal and other sources — into your diet. You'll watch the weight melt away in no time.

- Start your day with a bowl of whole-grain cereal or oatmeal for breakfast.
- Make sandwiches with whole-grain breads.
- Mix 3/4 cup of uncooked oats with each pound of ground beef or turkey when making meatballs, burgers, or meatloaf.
- Stir a handful of oats into your yogurt.

- Replace white rice with brown rice, barley, millet, buckwheat, bulgur, or quinoa.
- Add 1/2 cup of cooked wheat or rye berries, wild rice, brown rice, or barley to soups.
- Bake with half white flour and half whole-wheat flour.
- Grind oats in a food processor to make oat flour, and use it to make breads and pancakes.

'Whole' new reason to love popcorn

Munching on popcorn makes watching movies even more enjoyable. It can also make it much easier to fit into your pants. That's because popcorn and other whole grains may help reduce your waist size and zap belly fat.

Set your sights on three. Aim for at least three servings of whole grains, including popcorn, each day. In a study of 2,834 middle-aged Americans participating in the Framingham Heart Study, those who ate three or more servings of whole grains a day had 10 percent less visceral belly fat — the kind that surrounds your internal organs and boosts your risk of heart disease and diabetes — than those who ate virtually no whole grains. They also had significantly smaller waist sizes.

Popcorn was among the most common sources of whole grains in the study. One serving of air-popped popcorn is three cups.

Whole grains may help fight fat for a variety of reasons. They are rich in fiber, resistant starch, and oligosaccharides, and each could contribute by affecting appetite or insulin sensitivity. Whole grains also contain more vitamins, minerals, and phytochemicals than refined, or processed, grains.

But here's the catch. The beneficial link between whole grains and belly fat did not hold up for people whose diet also included at least four servings of refined grains. So that means just adding whole grains to your regular diet isn't enough. You need to swap refined grains for whole grains.

Besides popcorn, foods in the whole-grain category included whole-grain cold breakfast cereal, oatmeal, dark bread, brown rice, bran, wheat germ, and other grains like bulgur, kasha, and couscous.

White bread, English muffins, bagels, muffins, biscuits, pasta, pancakes, waffles, crackers, pizza, and many breakfast cereals are made with refined grains. Not surprisingly, white rice is a refined grain. Just snacking on popcorn rather than some of these foods could help make a difference.

Hold off hunger. Popcorn also trumps milk chocolate as a satisfying snack. A ConAgra Foods study found that women who ate a 100-calorie portion of popcorn felt more full than they did after eating chocolate nuggets with the same amount of calories. They also reported being more satisfied with the amount of food in their snack. As a filling, low-calorie, high-fiber snack, popcorn could play an important role in managing your weight. It should be noted that ConAgra makes Orville Redenbacher's popcorn.

Snack smartly. Of course, the health benefits of popcorn could be drowned with butter or smothered with salt. If you need to add some zip to your popcorn, try jazzing it up with garlic powder, curry powder, cayenne pepper, paprika, chili powder, or other spices.

One survey found that only 12 percent of Americans know that popcorn is a whole grain. But this kernel of wisdom can help you boost your whole-grain intake — and reduce your waist size.

Beat belly fat with blueberries

Stop feeling blue about your belly. Start eating more blueberries instead. You don't have to live with belly fat. Studies suggest that this fruit can trim your waist.

How do blueberries work their magic? They're packed with powerful polyphenols, including the anthocyanins that give them their dark blue color. Thanks to these plant chemicals, blueberries can help you achieve a flat belly.

Can't believe that there's a fruit that reduces belly fat? Read the surprising research.

Foil fat cells. A Texas Woman's University study found that blueberry polyphenols may thwart the development of fat cells. In this lab study, researchers added three doses of blueberry polyphenols to tissue taken from mice to measure the process by which a generic cell develops into a fat-storing cell.

Turns out this treatment decreased the formation of fat cells by up to 73 percent for the highest dose and 27 percent for the lowest. If further research confirms these results, adding blueberries to your diet could be an easy — and tasty — way to stop fat tissue from forming.

Banish belly fat. A University of Michigan study yielded similar results. Researchers fed lab rats either a low-fat or high-fat diet. They also mixed freeze-dried blueberry powder into both diets for half of the rats. Those who received the blueberry powder had less abdominal fat at the end of the 90-day study than those whose diets did not contain blueberry. They also had lower triglycerides and cholesterol and improved fasting glucose and insulin sensitivity — factors related to diabetes risk.

Slow down and focus to slim down

In a hurry to lose weight? Slow down. Chewing more can help you eat less. Chinese researchers found that obese people chewed less and ate more quickly than lean people. They also found that when you chew each bite 40 times rather than 15 times, you eat 12 percent less. Chewing more seems to affect the release of appetite-related hormones. It lowers levels of ghrelin, which stimulates hunger, and boosts levels of cholecystokinin, which curbs it.

Other research found that distracted eating — like gobbling dinner while watching TV — can prompt people to eat more. And it can lead to an increase in the snacks consumed later on. To manage your weight, don't use any electronics at mealtime. Walk away from your computer, turn off your tablet, put your phone away, and focus on your food. Set aside 20 minutes to do nothing but eat, and put your fork down between bites to savor your food.

The rats on the low-fat diet with blueberry powder saw the best results. They had lower body weight and a lower percentage of fat mass than the rats on the high-fat diet supplemented with blueberry powder.

These promising results suggest that blueberries can help battle obesity, as well as related conditions like heart disease and diabetes.

Increase your intake. In the meantime, feel free to add more blueberries to your diet. Toss some into your breakfast cereal or oatmeal, mix them into fruit salads, grab a handful for a snack, or just enjoy a bowl of blueberries for dessert. By adding more anthocyanin-rich blueberries to your diet, you just might subtract some belly fat.

Super sugar substitute

Sometimes the solution can be worse than the problem. Although you want to cut down on sugar, you don't want to replace it with a questionable artificial sweetener. Discover the one sugar substitute you don't have to worry about — sucralose.

Approved by the U.S. Food and Drug Administration (FDA) in 1998, sucralose appears in over 4,000 products, including dairy foods, cereals, desserts, baked goods, beverages, syrups, and condiments. Look for it on food labels. The most common brand name is Splenda. Sucralose is 600 times sweeter than sugar — so a little goes a long way.

In the past, other artificial sweeteners have been linked to cancer or mutations that can lead to cancer. Some may also come with unpleasant side effects, such as bloating, gas, or diarrhea. But to date, the FDA has not changed its stance on the safety of sucralose.

Use sucralose for cooking, baking, or just as a table sweetener. You'll get plenty of sweetness, but zero calories.

Trim your waistline with tea

Drinking more tea could be the key to losing belly fat. Studies suggest that this hot beverage reduces your waist size, fills you up, and fights fat. Find out how tea can help you achieve a flat belly.

Take two. A study found that men who drank 2 or more cups of tea a day had smaller waist circumferences than those who drank tea only occasionally or not at all. Oddly, the same link was not found for women.

Researchers at Queen's University in Canada tracked the drinking habits of 3,823 people who participated in the U.S. National

Health and Nutrition Examination Survey. While coffee had no effect on abdominal fat, frequent tea drinking did seem to help — at least for men.

What you put in your beverages might make a difference, too. Artificial sweeteners were linked to higher waist circumferences for both men and women. But men who added sugar and women who added milk to their coffee or tea had slimmer waist sizes.

Further research should shed more light on these potential links. But it can't hurt to boost your tea intake in the meantime.

Go green. Green tea gives you an edge in your battle with the scale. Dutch researchers who analyzed 11 studies involving green tea supplementation and weight loss determined that the catechins in green tea can significantly decrease body weight and help keep those extra pounds off.

In addition, Swedish researchers found that drinking green tea with a meal can make you feel more full and less likely to want to refill your plate with a second helping. Controlling your appetite could be one way green tea works its magic.

And a Thai study found that green tea helps your body burn more calories while resting and burn more fat overall, leading to a reduction in body weight.

Win with white. White tea, the least processed form of tea made from the buds and young leaves of the tea plant, also has fat-fighting properties. In lab studies, German scientists found that white tea extract breaks down human fat cells, while preventing new fat cells from forming. White tea may be so successful because it contains high concentrations of epigallocatechin-3-gallate and other polyphenols, as well as caffeine.

No matter what color tea you choose, you really can't go wrong. Just make sure to drink more of it. You'll find that sipping tea is a super way to slim down.

Fight fat with hot peppers

Heat up your weight loss efforts by sprinkling some cayenne pepper into your dishes. This fiery spice could decrease calorie intake, shrink fat tissue, and lower fat levels in the blood — so why not add more to your meals?

Cayenne and other spicy foods, like chili peppers and jalapenos, contain the compound capsaicin. Studies suggest that this red-hot substance fights weight gain in a variety of ways.

Curbs calories. Kick hunger to the curb by giving your meals an extra kick. A Purdue University study found that 1 gram, or 1/2 teaspoon, of cayenne pepper helped reduce hunger and burn more calories. Specifically, people had less desire to eat fatty, salty, or sweet foods. This effect on appetite was more pronounced in people who were not used to eating spicy foods, suggesting that it's possible to become desensitized to the heat.

> You may know that using smaller plates can trick you into eating smaller portions. But the color of your plates can also make a difference. Researchers found that people tend to give themselves more food if it blends into the plate — and less if there's a clear contrast in colors. For example, if you're dishing pasta with cream sauce onto a white plate, you'll give yourself more than if you served it on a red plate.

An earlier Dutch study reported similar results. People who received 0.9 grams of capsaicin 30 minutes before each meal felt more full and took in fewer calories and fat. The effect was greater in those who had their capsaicin mixed into their tomato juice rather than in pill form. The sensation of spiciness likely contributes to controlling hunger.

Unfortunately, this appetite-suppressing power may be short-lived. In a study of rats, those given capsaicin ate less at first, but after 10 days returned to their normal eating habits.

Zaps fat. Luckily, capsaicin does more than crush hunger — it also kills fat cells. That's what researchers in Taiwan discovered during lab studies. Capsaicin squashed the growth of fat cells and even triggered apoptosis, or cell death. It also reduced the amount of triglycerides and other lipids, or fats, within the cells.

Squelches inflammation. Obesity doesn't just mean extra weight — it means extra inflammation. South Korean researchers found that capsaicin clamps down on this inflammation by affecting the release of adipokines, molecules secreted from fat tissues or fat cells. Capsaicin suppresses inflammatory adipokines, while boosting levels of anti-inflammatory adiponectin. This double-barreled action not only guards against inflammation but also obesity-related complications such as diabetes and atherosclerosis, or hardening of the arteries.

Boosts metabolism. Rats on high-fat diets who also get capsaicin don't gain weight. It's not because they eat less, so something else must be going on. Capsaicin seems to interact with the TRPV1 receptor in your body to speed up metabolism and keep you from packing on the pounds. It's also possible capsaicin boosts calcium to help regulate the development of fat cells.

Another study shed more light on how capsaicin may help. In the study, rats who were fed capsaicin along with a high-fat diet lost 8 percent of their body weight. Turns out capsaicin triggers changes to 20 key proteins related to fat metabolism and burning calories.

However it works, capsaicin is worth a try. Aim for a teaspoon or two of cayenne or chili pepper a day, the amount found in a typical Indian or Thai diet. You'll find it's a spicy way to burn calories.

Amazing benefits from fish

Boost muscle, reduce fat, feel less fatigued, and have more energy — all with one amazing nutrient. If you like seafood, you'll be tickled pink.

That's because this fare contains a secret ingredient. It's astaxanthin, a carotenoid that gives salmon and lobster their pinkish color. Also found in trout, algae, and crustaceans like shrimp, krill, and crayfish, astaxanthin has emerged as a promising weapon against obesity in animal studies.

Boosts your metabolism. A high-fat diet puts you at high risk for obesity and related health problems. But astaxanthin may help counteract these pitfalls.

In a Japanese study, astaxanthin helped thwart weight gain and the accumulation of fatty tissue in mice fed a high-fat diet. The mice given astaxanthin also had less fatty livers and lower levels of triglycerides and cholesterol than mice fed a high-fat diet alone. Yet they didn't eat any less. It seems astaxanthin doesn't work by limiting calorie intake. Rather, it works by boosting metabolism so your body burns more energy — and more fat.

Revs up your workouts. Exercise plays an important role in any weight loss plan. Japanese researchers discovered that astaxanthin may make your workouts even more productive.

In a study of mice, astaxanthin boosted fat burning during exercise and improved muscle endurance. Specifically, mice treated with astaxanthin were able to run longer on a treadmill. Astaxanthin also helped speed up the loss of body fat that occurs with exercise.

Researchers note that astaxanthin promotes the burning of fat rather than glucose during exercise. But, as the previous study of mice on a high-fat diet suggests, astaxanthin may have a similar effect even when you're at rest.

In addition to these fat-burning benefits, astaxanthin has been studied for its antioxidant and anti-inflammatory properties. It may help people with rheumatoid arthritis, carpal tunnel syndrome, high cholesterol, vision problems, and other conditions. But evidence remains limited.

HEALTH ALERT!

About 1 in 4 Americans sit for more than eight hours a day. All those hours add up to nearly 122 days of sitting each year.

Sitting for an extended period of time can hurt your health — from waist size to blood sugar — even if you exercise. So use these tips to break your sedentary habits and add more movement into your day.

Break up your sitting with just one to three minutes of standing. Do this every half hour or so. Pace around while you're on the phone, or take the stairs instead of the elevator. If you're stuck somewhere where you can't stand, like the car, try fidgeting. Bounce your knees and tap your heels to get moving. You can also do some neck and shoulder stretches.

If you want to burn even more calories, try these creative ways to get more exercise every day. Shop in person instead of online, park farther away from the entrance when you go to the store, or clean your home.

Don't rush out to buy astaxanthin supplements. Wait until more studies — including human studies — demonstrate that these supplements are safe and effective.

In the meantime, feel free to get your astaxanthin the old-fashioned way — through your diet. Eating more seafood like salmon, shrimp, and lobster should do the trick. As a bonus, you'll reap the other established health benefits of fish. When choosing salmon, opt for Pacific sockeye salmon rather than farmed Atlantic salmon. You'll get about four times as much astaxanthin.

Lose pounds with legumes

In fairy tales, magic beans lead to towering beanstalks and adventures with giants. In reality, beans may not be magic — but they can be a giant help in your quest to lose weight.

A review examined the potential that beans and other legumes classified as pulses have for weight loss. A pulse is a type of legume harvested only for its dry grain. Pulses include peas, chickpeas, lentils, and dry beans like kidney beans, pinto beans, and navy beans but exclude peanuts and soybeans because they are also harvested for their oils.

The researchers found plenty of pluses for pulses. Here's a quick recap.

- Reduce the risk of obesity. In observational studies, people who ate more beans and other pulses were less likely to be obese. However, these kinds of studies do not prove cause and effect. Other diet and lifestyle factors may also play a role.
- Harness hunger. Some studies suggest that eating pulses can curb your appetite, at least temporarily. After eating pulses

rather than a control meal in one study, people tended to be less hungry and feel more full two to four hours later.

- Do more for your diet. Other studies show that adding pulses to your diet while also cutting back on total calories may help you lose even more weight.

More studies, especially long-term ones, are needed to confirm these positive results. But it makes sense that beans and other pulses would help. That's because they're packed with nutrients that contribute to feeling full and losing weight, including soluble and insoluble fiber, slowly digestible and resistant starches, protein, and phytochemicals.

Did you know?

You can become lighter just by eating a lighter lunch. When you limit calories at lunchtime, you don't necessarily compensate by eating more later in the day. That's what a Cornell University study discovered.

In the study, women chose foods from a buffet for their meals and snacks. After one week, roughly half of the women selected their lunch from six commercially available portion-controlled meals, while the others stuck to the buffet. For other meals and snacks, the women could eat as much as they wanted from the buffet. After two weeks, the groups switched their lunchtime tactics.

Researchers found that when women ate the portion-controlled lunches, they ate an average of 250 fewer calories each day and lost about a pound. Simply eating less at one meal can help you lose weight.

Unlike other valuable items, pulses don't come with a high price tag. In fact, beans rank among the cheapest — and most nutritious — foods out there. However, beans may cause bloating and excessive gas. Try reducing these unpleasant side effects by soaking dried beans for at least 16 hours before cooking.

Chances are you're not getting enough legumes in your diet, since most people fall far short of the U.S. Department of Agriculture's recommended amount. Most seniors age 60 and older should aim for 1 1/2 to 2 cups of this food — think beans, peas, and lentils — a week. Boosting your intake could be an easy way to lose weight. Give it a try. The pounds just might disappear — almost like magic.

Give hunger pangs the ax with flax

Flaxseed, thanks to its dietary fiber, may suppress your appetite. That's what Danish researchers discovered in a small study. The key seems to be mucilage, a type of soluble fiber found in flaxseed.

In the study, 18 young men were randomly given one of four meals containing varying amounts and sources of dietary fiber. Besides the control meal, one meal contained fiber from whole flaxseed, another featured low-mucilage flaxseed dietary fiber, and the last one included high-mucilage flaxseed dietary fiber.

The men who ate the high-mucilage flaxseed meal reported feeling more full than those who ate the control meal. The high-mucilage group also had much lower concentrations of lipids, or fats, in their blood. Both the mucilage groups had lower insulin levels compared to the other two groups. They also had a different response pattern to the hormone ghrelin, which stimulates hunger.

More research and larger studies are needed to confirm these results, but flaxseed could be a handy tool to curb your cravings. As a bonus, this food is an excellent source of heart-healthy omega-3 fatty acids.

In addition to squelching your appetite, flaxseed may fight high cholesterol, high blood pressure, heart disease, obesity, and cancer. Luckily, it's easy to sneak flaxseed into your diet. Just try these tricks.

- Sprinkle ground flaxseed on your cereal or oatmeal in the morning.
- Mix it into your batter for pancakes or waffles.
- Whip flaxseed into your smoothies.
- Stir ground flaxseed into your cottage cheese, applesauce, or yogurt.
- Add it to salads, soups, or rice pilaf.
- Use ground flaxseed in baked goods like breads, muffins, and cookies.
- Mix it into meatloaf, casseroles, and burgers.
- Replace fat in recipes with flaxseed. Swap 3 tablespoons of ground flaxseed for 1 tablespoon of shortening, butter, margarine, or oil.

Simple way to slim down

Here's a refreshing — and refreshingly simple — way to lose weight. Drink more water. Studies show that drinking water before meals or in place of other beverages can help you cut calories and peel off the pounds. Find out how water can make a big splash in your diet.

Drink and shrink. Water fills you up, but it doesn't have any calories. That makes it the perfect pre-meal beverage. If you feel more full, you'll eat less during the following meal.

Virginia Tech researchers found that dieters who drink water before meals lose more weight than those who don't. In the study, which included 48 people ages 55 to 75, those who drank 2 cups of water before meals lost more weight than those who didn't. The water drinkers lost about 15.5 pounds during the 12-week study, while the others shed about 11 pounds. Both groups were on a low-calorie diet.

An earlier study by the same researchers showed that drinking 2 cups of water before a meal resulted in eating 75 to 90 fewer calories during that meal. Those calories can add up to a big drop in numbers on the scale.

It may not even take 2 cups of water to blunt your appetite. A Vanderbilt University study discovered that drinking a little more than 1/2 cup — 4.5 ounces — of water 20 minutes before each meal helps boost feelings of fullness.

Researchers compared the effects of whole grapefruit, grapefruit juice, and water. Turns out water worked just as well as grapefruit to curb calories and promote weight loss. In fact, the water drinkers lost 15 pounds in 12 weeks.

Swap the soda pop. Drink water instead of sugary drinks, and you'll reap even more benefits. You'll still quench your thirst, but you won't swallow empty calories. This simple switch can make a big difference. In fact, researchers in one weight-loss study estimated that overweight female dieters could lose 5 pounds and shrink their waist size by an inch if they simply replaced 80 percent of their sweetened drinks with water.

Skipping sweet drinks has other health benefits as well. Another study found that women who drank two or more sugary drinks a day increased their risk of heart disease and diabetes. Their waistlines also expanded — even if they didn't gain weight.

Did you know?

Is muscle pain keeping you from playing all 18 holes? If so, you'll want to take note of a solution that will let you play golf pain-free.

For starters, you'll want to warm up before each game. Start with a light activity — a five- to 10-minute walk is an excellent option. Then you'll want do some stretches.

You can begin by bending over and touching your toes. This loosens your hamstrings and releases tension in your lower back. Then focus on your hips. Seated in a chair, place your right ankle on top of your left knee. Push down on your right knee, and lean forward until you feel a gentle pull in your hip. Repeat on the opposite side.

Lastly, stretch your wrist muscles. With your palm facing down, hold your right arm in front of you. Gently pull your wrist up by grabbing the tops of your fingers with your left hand. Repeat with your left arm.

When you're off the course, add strength training to your exercise routine. Soon you'll be teeing off like a pro. That's because strength training helps you build muscle mass and lose fat.

Pour some more. Increase your water intake, and decrease your weight. Researchers found that drinking a little more than a quart of water each day helped overweight female dieters lose more weight regardless of which diet they followed or how much exercise they got. Water may even promote fat oxidation, or the burning of fat, both when you're exercising and at rest.

Try drinking water before meals, in place of caloric drinks, and throughout the day. Consider carrying a water bottle so you'll always have some on hand. If plain water seems too boring, jazz it up by dropping some berries into your glass.

Drinking water might just be the easiest way to lose weight — zero calories, zero costs, zero problems.

Turn ugly flab into rock-hard abs

You don't need to do hundreds of gut-wrenching sit ups and crunches to strengthen your core. Instead, you can flatten your stomach with a gentle and easy workout called the modified plank. Here's how.

Lie on your stomach and raise yourself up so that you're resting on your forearms and knees. Tighten your abdominal muscles by pushing your navel toward your spine. Hold this pose for three to five seconds. Then return to your original position and repeat.

Wounds & injuries

Heal with honey, inside and out

Ancient Egyptians and Greeks knew it. In fact, Aristotle called it a good salve for wounds. Science is finally catching up and finding that honey really can help wounds heal faster.

- Honey draws lymph from your body into the wound, flushing out bacteria and dirt.
- Its natural acidity creates the ideal conditions for your body to repair the wound.
- It protects wounds by blocking the growth of certain bacteria, including *Escherichia (E.) coli*, *Staphylococcus aureus* (staph), and even methicillin-resistant *S. aureus*, better known as the drug-resistant bug MRSA.
- Bandages that contain honey help your body form new skin over the top of the wound, protecting it.

All in all, studies show honey can help these types of injuries heal more quickly, and with less scarring. And research suggests it can even help clear up chronically infected wounds.

Go for the gold. The best honey for wound healing may be manuka, a variety made from the nectar of the manuka tree in Australia and New Zealand. Studies show it can block the growth of 80 different types of bacteria. One type, *Streptococcus pyogenes*, is often the cause of wounds that won't heal.

This type of bacteria infects the wound and clumps together to form a film that can prevent antibiotics from reaching the injury and helping it heal. British researchers discovered that manuka honey killed up to 85 percent of these bacteria and kept them from forming this film.

Get better inside. Honey heals from the inside, too. Eating honey reduces disease-causing inflammation in your body by lowering levels of prostaglandins, inflammation-causing compounds. It also acts as a prebiotic, which naturally boosts your immune system.

Know what to buy. Store-bought honey won't necessarily provide benefits like these. It has been heat-treated to keep it from fermenting. Unfortunately, heat can destroy some of honey's natural healing properties. Raw, unprocessed honey, however, may not be safe. It could actually worsen an infection if it's contaminated with *C. botulinum* or other organisms.

Herbal cure for open wounds

Which herb has the most antioxidant healing power? Three varieties of one common spice took first, second, and third place — and it wasn't garlic. Amazingly, oregano beat out 27 other cooking herbs in one study. Mexican oregano, Italian oregano, and Greek mountain oregano took the top three spots.

No one recommends rubbing oregano into a cut to help it heal. However, scientists have managed to make an ointment containing oregano extract that:

- fights infection.
- helps minimize scarring.
- blocks the growth of dangerous bacteria like MRSA.
- kills other infection-causing bugs.

Look for this specialized salve on store shelves in the future.

Find the middle ground. Look for locally made, raw, filtered honey. Filtering removes impurities and makes it more sterile. Or order a jar of manuka honey, the kind used in many studies, from Comvita through its website *comvita.com*. This company also produces Medihoney, a medical-grade honey approved for use by the U.S. Food & Drug Administration. You can buy manuka-infused Medihoney antibacterial wound gel online.

CLA mends cuts quicker

A little-known fat in milk and meat could help wounds heal faster. Some animals, like cows and sheep, have a rumen. It's a special part of their stomach that breaks down tough plants such as grass. Here, bacteria go to work. They help the animal digest this plant material by fermenting it first. This produces conjugated linoleic acid (CLA), an unsaturated fat that makes its way into milk, cheese, eggs, and the meat from cows and sheep.

Controls inflammation. Scientists say that CLA speeds up an early stage of healing that's known as the inflammatory stage. This period is key to healing successfully.

It's when immune system cells such as macrophages and neutrophils flood the wound, attacking harmful germs and cleaning out debris. They pump out large amounts of reactive oxygen species (ROS). These compounds guard the injury against bacteria.

ROS are a double-edged sword. In the right amounts, they help wounds heal. But too much of them for too long can slow down the healing process. Sometimes immune cells produce too much ROS.

That's where CLA steps in. It douses ROS and turns down the volume on inflammation, so it doesn't go on for too long. That, in turn, may help wounds mend more quickly.

Speeds healing. It seems to have worked for mice. Mice with open wounds healed faster when CLA was added to their food. This fat calmed inflammation around the injuries and helped those wounds close more rapidly.

Milk and lamb offer the most CLA, followed by beef and veal. But buyer beware — what cows and sheep eat has a huge impact on the CLA content that you'll find in these foods. For example, grass-fed cattle produce milk with five times more CLA, plus have five-and-a-half times more CLA in their meat than cattle fed a typical high-grain diet.

CLA is found in the fat of dairy foods, so nonfat and low-fat dairy products don't provide much of this compound. Of course, it's not healthy to load up on high-fat foods just to help a cut heal faster. Always eat full-fat dairy and red meat in moderation.

> A spoonful of sugar does more than help medicine go down. It can soothe a burned tongue. Simply stick your tongue directly against the sugar. As the granules dissolve, they will pull heat away from your tongue.

Seafood helps wounds heal

Arginine, an amino acid your body uses to build proteins, plays a major role in healing wounds. Your body turns arginine into two key compounds.

In the first two or three days of healing, it turns arginine into nitric oxide. This compound widens blood vessels to increase blood flow to injured areas and prevents the growth of bacteria.

After that, your body switches gears, turning arginine into ornithine. This compound helps grow new cells and form collagen, the fibers that knit skin back together.

Many studies show that getting extra arginine boosts the formation of collagen and strengthens the new tissue that forms. This makes wounds less likely to reopen. In addition, it may help heal cuts, like those from surgery.

Ample arginine is especially important if you have diabetes or take corticosteroids. People with diabetes don't produce as much nitric oxide around their injuries. Perhaps as a result, their bodies tend to form less collagen around wounds, and their wounds break open more easily. Getting more arginine may bring nitric oxide and collagen levels back to normal, according to animal studies.

Corticosteroids, on the other hand, are linked to lower levels of inducible nitric oxide synthase (iNOS) around injuries. The enzyme iNOS helps build nitric oxide. It's no surprise, then, that these drugs may keep wounds from healing properly.

Arginine is easy to get from a wide range of foods, but crunchy crustaceans like shrimp, crab, and lobster top the list. For every 200 calories you eat of:

- canned blue crab, you net 4.2 grams (g) of arginine.
- cooked lobster, there's 3.9 g.
- cooked shrimp, you get 3.8 g of arginine.
- cooked crayfish, Dungeness crab, and Alaskan king crab, there's more than 3 g of arginine apiece.

Not a big fan of seafood? Try turkey. These gobblers give you 2 g in a 200-calorie serving of roasted white meat. Vegans can make certain they get adequate arginine by munching on cooked spinach or dried seaweed, otherwise known as spirulina.

Sunburn protection in a cup

Drinking green tea may protect your skin from sunburn. This ancient beverage is loaded with flavonoids, powerful plant compounds that guard your body against all sorts of diseases.

In nature, plants use these compounds to protect themselves from sun damage. Flavonoids absorb ultraviolet light. It makes sense that they could offer similar protection in people.

Sixty middle-age women tested the power of green tea antioxidants against the sun's ultraviolet rays. Half drank a beverage enriched with green tea antioxidants each day for 12 weeks. The other half drank a beverage made to look and taste like the real thing but with no actual green tea.

The women were exposed to ultraviolet rays at the beginning of the study and again at the end. Researchers measured their sunburn each time. At the end of 12 weeks, UV-induced skin redness decreased by 25% among the green tea drinkers.

All of that green tea boosted the amount of blood and oxygen that reached skin cells. The result, scientists say — the women's skin became less sensitive to damaging UV rays, and became smoother, more elastic, and less scaly.

Did you know?

Stop the itching from poison ivy fast with this easy treatment. Simply soak a clean rag in cold, whole milk. Wring it out, and leave the damp rag on your rash for 10 to 15 minutes. Then rinse off the milk with warm water.

Index

A

B

C

D

E

F

H

I

N

O

P

Q

R

S

T